DR. COLBERT'S
Spiritual
HEALTH ZONE

DON COLBERT, MD

SILOAM

Cataloging-in-Publication Data is on file with the Library of Congress.
International Standard Book Number: 978-1-63641-256-6
E-book ISBN: 978-1-63641-257-3

1 2024
Printed in the United States of America

Most Charisma Media products are available at special quantity discounts for bulk purchase for sales promotions, premiums, fund-raising, and educational needs. For details, call us at (407) 333-0600 or visit our website at www.charismamedia.com.

This book is dedicated to my seven grandchildren, Braden, Dylan, Timothy, Caleb, Jaret, Kate, and Olen. Thank God that they are all born again, but I also pray that each one will be a bright light in a dark world, and that each one will let their light shine and bring multitudes into the kingdom of God.

We are living in dark times, and evil is increasing, as prophesied in Isaiah 5:20: "Woe to those who call evil good, and good evil; who put darkness for light, and light for darkness."

I am amazed at how filth, pornography, lying, cheating, stealing, and immorality are accepted now as the norm. The key to life is simply walking and living in the love of God, and letting that love shine and flow out to a sick and dying world by the Holy Spirit, "because the love of God has been poured out in our hearts by the Holy Spirit who was given to us" (Rom. 5:5). And by this love "all will know that you are My disciples, if you have love for one another" (John 13:35, emphasis added).

CONTENTS

THE GREAT FALLING AWAY

M ANY PEOPLE STUDY the future for a variety of reasons: to make money, to plan for crises, to strategize how to evangelize the world for Jesus. But from a strictly medical point of view, the coming last days of this age will witness the worst health conditions ever experienced on planet Earth. The good news is that as believers in Christ, we don't need to suffer any of these afflictions—if we abide in love as God commands us to do. That is the purpose of this book: to show practically how to maximize our health in body, mind, and soul by living out the love walk.

The Bible tells us we are headed into a time when not only societies and governments will be shaken but physical and mental wellness as well. Human beings will come under great pressure. I believe we are already in such days. But God has given us the key to divine health, and this key never fails. Whatever you believe about Christians being present on the earth for any part of the perilous times and tribulations, one thing is certain: God has not appointed His children ever to suffer as the world does, in any generation. We are called instead to walk in fullness of life—and this we can do confidently if we bring our actions, words, and thoughts into alignment with the foundational principle of God's kingdom: love.

THE RISE OF WOKE CHRISTIANITY

Without being anchored to love, some disaffected Christians are turning to religions such as Islam, Hinduism, or Buddhism. George Barna's research shows a startling growth of Islam in America from a footnote statistic a few decades ago to "a significant faith group" today. "Right now, in America, it appears that the number of Muslims here outnumber how many Jews we have in America," he said.[1]

There is also a rise in antisemitism in the world at the writing of this book. Other Americans, especially millennials, are turning away from established religion altogether, with 43 percent saying they don't believe or know if God exists. Barna describes their worldview as based on "the universal purpose of life of being happy and feeling good about oneself." They "reject biblical principles in favor of more worldly spiritual perspectives and practices."[2]

IT'S A FACT!

Millennials express skepticism of established religion, and 43 percent say they don't know if God exists. George Barna reports they "reject biblical principles in favor of more worldly spiritual perspectives and practices."[3]

Jesus preached both the love of the Father and repentance, which means turning from our sins. Matthew 4:17 reads, "From that time Jesus began to preach and to say, 'Repent, for the kingdom of heaven is at hand.'" Paul wrote in 1 Timothy 4:1–2 (AMP), "But the [Holy] Spirit explicitly and unmistakably declares that in later times some will turn away from the faith, paying attention instead to deceitful and seductive spirits and doctrines of demons, [misled] by the hypocrisy of liars whose consciences are seared as with a branding iron [leaving them incapable of ethical functioning]."

The woke church offers loveless versions of biblical principles such as justice, mercy, and love. But the only power they possess is of coercion with methods such as cancellation, threats of job loss, loss of friends, reputation, and so on. The tragedy is that woke Christianity is leading many sincere believers astray from the true faith. Jesus talked about such people in the parable of the soils. They receive the seed of His Word enthusiastically but fail to bear fruit because of the pleasures, riches, and cares of life. They become acquisitive rather than generous. They seek fun and money rather than righteousness. I believe the love of many Christians is being choked by things of this world—with the encouragement of so-called church "leaders." They ignore that 1 John 2:15 (KJV) says, "Love not the world, neither the things that are in the world. If any man love the world, the love of the Father is not in him."

We must be honest with ourselves and ask, How much has the "affirming" quasi-gospel of woke Christianity affected and infected our own hearts? Probably more than we think. Ask yourself, Why is it that most Christians do not walk in more love, peace, or power? Where is our joy, gentleness, faith, patience, and other fruit of the Spirit? Why are so many believers anxious, depressed, greedy, and self-centered?

IT'S A FACT!

"Despite rising inflation, America's appetite for luxury goods has increased dramatically over the past four years, with 86% more Americans in-market for luxury items than in 2021."[4] Common luxury items include expensive cars, timepieces (watches), jewelry, designer clothing, yachts, corporate helicopters, private jets, large residences, urban mansions, and country homes.

The obvious answer is that we have lost the love of God. When we love the pleasures, positions, and purposes of the world around us, we unplug from the life of God and grow unhealthy in our minds, souls, and bodies. His life within us is choked out. Today, many Christians resemble the description found in 2 Timothy 3:5 (KJV), "having a form of godliness, but denying the power thereof." For this reason, they are also unhealthy in mind and body.

This is why John warned soberly in 1 John 2:15–17, "Do not love the world or the things in the world. If anyone loves the world, the love of the Father is not in him. For all that is in the world—the lust of the flesh, the lust of the eyes, and the pride of life—is not of the Father but is of the world. And the world is passing away, and the lust of it; but he who does the will of God abides forever."

When we love the world, we put ourselves on the pathway to death because, as John put it, "the world is passing away." Before we proceed, take a moment to consider, What is your condition? What do you love most? What do you spend your time, money, and thoughts on? What are you looking forward to in life? Retirement? Your next vacation? Sports or entertainment events? Your next meal? These are all blessings, but they become idols when they take the top spots in our affections. They easily become the pleasures of the world Jesus warned about.

If Jesus is Lord of your life, He will have something to say about the movies or TV shows you watch, the friends you fellowship with, and every word that proceeds out of your mouth.

If He is Lord of your life, He will have something to say about where you go online, what apps you use, and the comments and posts you make on social media.

If He is Lord of your life, He will have something to say about your finances—how you make your money, how you spend your money, and where you give your money.

If He is Lord of your life, He will have something to say about what you eat and how you take care of your body.

If He is Lord of your life, He will have something to say about who you date and who you marry, how you treat your spouse, and how you raise your children.

If He is Lord of your life, He will have something to say about the atmosphere of your home, the music you listen to, the words you speak, and the way you steward your own emotions.

If He is Lord of your life, He wants to rule over every area of your life. As Paul pleaded,

> I beseech you therefore, brethren, by the mercies of God, that you present your bodies a living sacrifice, holy, acceptable to God, which is your reasonable service. And do not be conformed to this world, but be transformed by the renewing of your mind, that you may prove what is that good and acceptable and perfect will of God.
>
> —ROMANS 12:1–2

WALKING IN DIVINE HEALTH IN THE END TIMES

God's plan for believers in all times is that we walk in greater and greater health, even if we are present on earth during the great falling away. The Bible indicates many times that when things worsen around us, Christians only grow brighter and stronger. Paul said that when the culture around us becomes crooked and perverse, Jesus' followers "shine as lights in the world" (Phil. 2:15). When early Christian martyr Stephen was persecuted, "all who sat in the council, looking steadfastly at him, saw his face as the face of an angel" (Acts 6:15). And when three righteous Hebrews—Shadrach, Meshach, and Abednego— were thrown into the fiery furnace for refusing to bow down to an idol, a fourth man appeared with them, "and they are not hurt, and the form of the fourth is like the Son of God," said King Nebuchadnezzar, who was looking on (Dan. 3:25). "And the satraps, administrators, governors, and the king's counselors gathered together, and they saw these men on whose bodies the fire had no power; the hair of their head was not singed nor were their garments affected, and the smell of fire was not on them" (v. 27).

Even in the fire these men remained perfectly healthy.

God's love imparts not only spiritual health but the highest level of physical and mental health. Not everyone will endure persecution without a scratch as Shadrach, Meshach, and Abednego did, but for believers who walk in love with Jesus and others, wellness will actually accelerate as we near the end of the age. In a famous passage, Paul wrote beautifully about how believers act and speak in the power of God's love. "Therefore, since we have such hope, we use great boldness of speech," he began, indicating a vibrancy and robustness inside and out (2 Cor. 3:12).

He continued a few verses later, "Now the Lord is the Spirit; and where the Spirit of the Lord is, there is liberty" (v. 17). Christians usually spiritualize this verse to mean liberty in worship, but this liberty is all-encompassing and includes things like freedom of physical movement, facility of thought, and freedom from emotional or mental shackles or weights. Paul then added, "But we all, with unveiled face, beholding as in a mirror the glory of the Lord, *are being transformed into the same image from glory to glory, just as by the Spirit of the Lord*" (v. 18, emphasis added).

How amazing is that? As we walk "by the Spirit" we go "from glory to glory." This is why the writer of Hebrews could confidently encourage us, "Let us run with endurance the race that is set before us, looking unto Jesus" (Heb. 12:1–2). While others are falling apart, love-fueled believers will be running at marathon levels!

While darkness and dysfunction may increase, light and glory will always increase for those who accept God's love. We will again see days like those of Charles Finney, when entire cities were converted through his revival meetings. We will see outpourings of the Spirit like the ones described in the Book of Acts, but they will be happening all over the globe at the same time. Nothing in all of history can compare to the move of God that will come upon the earth in those last days for all who will receive it—and this revival will include top levels of physical and mental health.

Right now the best thing we can do for our minds, bodies, and souls is learn to walk in the empowering, cleansing, strengthening love of God. This will protect us from disease and promote all aspects of health. Let me begin by telling the story of how I came to a life-changing moment of revelation about God's love—the source of all health, which has the power to transform your life in every way.

SECTION I:
THE SOURCE OF DIVINE HEALTH

CHAPTER 1

MY LOVE REVOLUTION

M Y EPIPHANY DIDN'T happen on the road to Damascus, but what I experienced one morning three years ago changed my life and medical practice, casting a big, bright light on the true source of all health for body, mind, and soul. The revelation I received that day became the most important one in my forty-plus years as a doctor.

The day began quietly in the kitchen where I was brewing up some good coffee and listening to one of my favorite sermons. I like to wake up early and dive straight into the Word of God, either turning on an audio version of the Bible or finding a good message by a Spirit-filled preacher. Years ago I gave up blasting myself with the news every morning because it only tends to breed anxiety and put my mind on the wrong things. I need to anchor my thoughts to Jesus and eternal realities, which are far more powerful and enduring than whatever is swirling around in the latest news cycle. Plus, the Bible says the Lord will keep our minds in perfect peace when we set our minds on Him (Isa. 26:3), and the news is anything but peaceful.

On this particular morning I chose to listen to a message on the subject of love by Kenneth Hagin, Sr. In it Hagin stated that far too many believers have made Jesus their Savior from hell but not the Lord of their lives. Love, he said, is the main message of the gospel but not the main focus of most believers' lives.

That's when it hit me. For some reason his words stopped me in my tracks. I realized in a burst of insight that as a medical professional, operating a practice and writing more than fifty books during my career, I had helped people find health and freedom through better eating habits, exercise, lowering their blood pressure, taking the right supplements, having good thought practices, and more—but love had never been central to my approach. Of all the life-enhancing topics I had researched and taught, somehow I had never emphasized the core message of the gospel: love.

How could I have missed it, I thought, as the magnitude of the revelation sank in. How could I have dealt with so many matters of health and wellness in such a detailed way, yet mostly given peripheral attention to their Source? In some ways I had been examining the branches of health while ignoring the tree trunk—or, more accurately, ignoring the root. As the supreme characteristic of God and the number one goal of all His children, love should have formed the foundation of my work from the beginning.

I stood in the kitchen, totally taken off guard by the flood of new ideas. I realized I had climbed to the top of the health and wellness field and missed the main thing. Without discounting the good that God in His grace had allowed me to do, I had to admit I had leaned heavily on my intellect and not on issues of the heart. I had emphasized the physical aspects of care while addressing the deeper root causes with a fairly light hand.

Please don't get me wrong; basic health and wellness are a crucial and valuable part of God's plan for each one of us, but no matter how well we achieve optimum fitness and nutrition, these bodies of ours all have expiration dates. For most people it happens when we are around eighty years old. Then, no matter how well we have cared for our bodies, they go into the grave while our spirits, as believers, go to heaven, where we give account for everything we did on earth. Which is more important: how well we ate, exercised, and optimized our hormones, or how well we loved? The answer now seemed obvious to me.

IT'S A FACT!

The 2022 life expectancy for men in the United States was 74.8 years; the life expectancy for women was 80.2 years. For both sexes, expected lifespan averaged 77.5 years.[1]

Just as important to me as a doctor, I realized that as the crowning characteristic of God Himself, love had to be the very best thing for the body and mind, not just the spirit. This wasn't theoretical; it had to be a scientific fact.

While I had done my best to keep people alive longer and with greater energy and effectiveness in life, I had not put their attention on the wellspring of all health—which perhaps explained why I was so frequently bothered by the number of patients I had seen through the years who called themselves Christians but didn't walk consistently in the abundant life of God. Yes, their health improved with my treatments and their lifestyle changes, but many patients also seemed to hit a ceiling. Though I helped them with the things doctors can do—lowering blood pressure, improving heart health, and more—they still seemed to fall short of thriving in Christ as the Bible promises we will do. Like me, they were spending a lot of time focusing on the minors and not the majors. The biggest major of them all is the love walk; that is, abiding in the love of God and learning to love God, ourselves, and others with all our strength, which also includes forgiving ourselves and others.

I have to emphasize it again so nobody gets me wrong: Medical knowledge is incredibly valuable and has done immeasurable good in the world. So have advances in psychology, nutrition, and so forth. But all human knowledge pales in the presence of love, which is God's ultimate attribute. The Bible clearly states that knowledge is limited and can even be deceiving. Paul wrote that knowledge will pass away, lose its value, and be superseded by love (1 Cor. 13:8, 13). Love, he reminded us, goes on forever. He also pointed out—painfully to some of us—that knowledge causes people to be puffed up, while love helps people to be built up (1 Cor. 8:1). Knowledge alone cannot and will not take people to a place of optimum health in their bodies, minds, and emotions. Only love, the eternal, nourishing root of all wellness, can do that. Medical knowledge and health principles work and are totally valid, but as Paul said, there is a "more excellent way," which is love.

WHAT IS LOVE?

As I studied love more deeply, I was struck over and over by love's profundity and practicality. It is completely inexhaustible, imminently powerful, and easily obtainable. Yet we have dumbed down love to mean little more than a feeling, a passing desire, an affection based in our own sentiments, whims, or emotions. We have limited it to a strong attachment when in fact it is the sustaining force of all existence. The Bible says God is love (1 John 4:8)—and it is impossible to overstate the magnitude of that statement. There is no greater power in heaven or earth than love.

Unfortunately, we often throw the word around like it's cheap.

"I love football."

"I love ice cream."

"I love my new car."

"I love that person."

"I love a good movie."

"I love jewelry."

We would be wise to heed John the apostle's words when he wrote, as we saw earlier:

> Do not love the world or the things in the world. If anyone loves the world, the love of the Father is not in him. For all that is in the world—the lust of the flesh, the lust of the eyes, and the pride of life—is not of the Father but is of the world.
>
> —1 JOHN 2:15–16

Love is not a feeling or a special inclination. Rather, "God is love, and he who abides in love abides in God, and God in him" (1 John 4:16).

God loves us with an everlasting love, wrote Jeremiah the prophet:

> The LORD has appeared of old to me, saying: "Yes, I have loved you with an everlasting love; therefore with lovingkindness I have drawn you."
>
> —JEREMIAH 31:3

As Christians, we do not have the option of relegating love to second place. Jesus said in John 13:34–35 (KJV):

> A new commandment I give unto you [not a suggestion or consideration], that ye love one another; as I have loved you, that ye also love one another. By this shall all men know that ye are my disciples, if ye have love one to another.

In Matthew 22:36–40 a lawyer asked Jesus,

> "Teacher, which is the great commandment in the law?" Jesus said to him, "'You shall love the LORD your God with all your heart, with all your soul, and with all your mind.' This is the first and great commandment. And the second is like it: 'You shall love your neighbor as yourself.' On these two commandments hang all the Law and the Prophets."

But a few days later Jesus gave His followers a new commandment: to love one another as Jesus loves us (John 13:34). This love can only be attained by the new birth and the Holy Spirit because the love of God has been shed abroad in our hearts by the Holy Spirit (Rom. 5:5, KJV). That kind of love is a sign of our faith and unmistakably marks the life of a believer. Without it, the world will not even know we are Christians.

In his book *The Four Loves*, C. S. Lewis identified the four primary types of love, based on the following Greek words:

- Eros—passion, lust, sexual attraction, and physical love
- Phileo—friendship love, the kind shared between close family members and friends, characterized by trust and loyalty

- Storge—parental love for children; protective and in many ways selfless, like the love of a mother for her child
- Agape—God's kind of love; compassionate and empathetic, especially toward the weak and down-and-out. It is unselfish and expects nothing in return.

The love Jesus spoke of is agape love and transcends even our human attempts to define it. It is the essence of a perfect God who gives us His affections, attention, and eternal blessings in spite of how badly we sometimes treat Him. So the apostle John wrote:

> Beloved, let us love one another: for love is of God; and every one that loveth is born of God, and knoweth God. He that loveth not knoweth not God; for God is love.... Beloved, if God so loved us, we ought also to love one another.
>
> —1 JOHN 4:7–8, 11, KJV

And,

> We have known and believed the love that God has for us.
>
> —1 JOHN 4:16

> God is love; and he that dwelleth in love dwelleth in God, and God in him. Herein is our love made perfect, that we may have boldness in the day of judgment: because as he is, so are we in this world. There is no fear in love; but perfect love casteth out fear.
>
> —1 JOHN 4:16–18, KJV

The sobering truth is that love is the single sign that you and I are walking with the Lord. John wrote:

> We know that we have passed from death [spiritual death] unto life [everlasting life], because we love the brethren. He that loveth not his brother abideth in death. Whosoever hateth his brother is a murderer: and ye know that no murderer hath eternal life abiding in him.
> —1 John 3:14–15, KJV

A Change of Direction

Maybe you've come to a crossroads of your own before. Maybe you've even hit a dead end where it seemed there was nowhere left to go. Or maybe, like me, you've had a life-transforming moment of insight. We probably all need a strong jolt to change our minds at times. Saul of Tarsus famously experienced a world-altering one-eighty on that road to Damascus. He was the cream of the religious crop of his day, ascending to the apex of intellectual and religious achievement. Yet his mind totally changed in a moment of time when Jesus forcibly interrupted him on his way to persecute Christians in Syria. (See Acts 9.) Saul became physically blind for several days, even fasting from food and water until Ananias, a godly man, prayed for him and gave him a message with guidance from the Lord.

Notice how Saul's physical health was impacted by his interaction with Jesus. I believe this is always the case, though not always so dramatic. It took Saul—now called Paul—a while to absorb this new revelation. He went into the desert of Arabia for a period of years to consider the seismic shift that had taken place in his mind and heart after that stunning encounter.

We too can benefit from "suddenly" moments of God. They help us to renew our minds in Christ Jesus, to move from consuming only the "milk" of the Word to eating meat. (See 1 Corinthians 3:1–3.) This is not to say that everything that came before in our lives is bad. All babies need milk before they can handle meat. Even Paul was operating in a form of God-given revelation before meeting Jesus—but then a better revelation showed up. He was following the Law of Moses, which Jesus supported, but then Jesus established a new covenant and Paul had to change his mind. The old way of the law wasn't going to work anymore. Paul didn't abandon the Old Testament when he came to believe in Jesus, but he did have to study and understand it in a fresh light.

So it was for me, and so it is for many of you. We must allow Jesus to reshape our notions of what is best for the health of our bodies, minds, and souls. Then we need to do as Paul did and recenter our lives around God's love.

My "Suddenly" Moment

That morning, it struck me with heavenly force that I needed to journey further upstream to the headwaters of health from which all other remedies flow. I could take people higher, helping them to truly thrive in body and soul. But in my frail humanity, I was afraid to try. I had become proficient at helping people achieve their health goals in ways that were by now very familiar to me. I was at the top of my game professionally, but I also knew something critical was missing, and so I gave myself no choice but to obey what I knew to be a heavenly revelation.

"Lord, forgive me for overlooking the greatest source of life and health there is," I prayed that morning. "The truth is I'm not a preacher; I'm a medical doctor. I don't know how to help people take the love walk, but I will step out in faith and do my best. From here on, in my medical practice and with my books,

I will help people obtain and implement the most important thing in Your kingdom: love."

When I made up my mind to major on love and minor on everything else, believing that by putting it in its proper place everything else would follow, it didn't take long to see amazing results. Instead of treating symptoms and even physical causes of disease and discomfort, I now aimed for the root causes of people's problems. I watched as patients truly became free by embracing the biblical mandate to walk in God's love, which has so many ramifications for our behavior, thoughts, and words. Soon I was even leading people to the Lord in my own office, employees included!

After three years my practice—not to mention my own life— was revolutionized. I now see that love is the key to all types of health—physical, emotional, and mental. Nothing else can replace it or duplicate its power to heal. This is not theory or mere teaching. I watch day after day as love transforms lives and marriages. I see how abiding in love

- makes us more resistant to disease;
- helps to lengthen our lives by removing deadly habits, thoughts, and emotions;
- vastly improves our experience of life as pleasurable, purposeful, and eternally significant;
- helps to reset the stress response, enabling us to live in peace and joy; and
- heals relationships.

A study titled "Love Promotes Health" found that love most definitely impacts our health and well-being. "The better we understand the concrete neurobiology of love and its possible secondary implications, the greater is our respect for the significance and potency of love's role in mental and physical health....Love, compassion and joy make our immune system function better and help to battle diseases."[2]

Research repeatedly shows that people whose lives are marked by the giving and receiving of love—with meaningful close relationships—"are happier and healthier than people with less love in their lives....Perhaps the best example of this comes from Harvard researchers who followed a group of men for over 80 years of their lives. The researchers found that warm and loving close relationships, whether with friends, family, or spouses, were among the best predictors of well-being across the entire lifespan."[3]

In fact, the very biochemistry of love impacts your body and well-being in ways we never previously imagined. Researchers have discovered that "the molecules associated with love have restorative properties, including the ability to literally heal a 'broken heart.'...Oxytocin [one of these molecules] can facilitate adult neurogenesis and tissue repair, especially after a stressful experience....The heart seems to rely on oxytocin as part of a normal process of protection and self-healing."[4]

IT'S A FACT!

Men are four times more likely than women to report watching pornography in the past month. Fifty-seven percent of men ages thirty to forty-nine report having watched pornography in the past month. Viewing pornography is associated with high rates of loneliness, feelings of dissatisfaction with personal appearance, insecurity, and feeling less satisfied with one's sex life.[5]

A review of one major aspect of love—the presence of healthy social relationships—found that "the quality and quantity of our relationships influences our risk of dying as much as other well-established risk factors for mortality, such as smoking and alcohol consumption, and exceeds the influence of other risk factors such as physical inactivity and obesity"![6]

Looking at nearly 150 studies with more than three hundred thousand participants, the researchers concluded that there is a 50 percent increased likelihood of survival for people with meaningful social relationships. This finding remained consistent regardless of age, sex, initial health status, and other factors. Participants who lived with others and had strong networks of friends and community members were less likely to die compared to those who, for example, lived alone and had a less-robust social life.[7]

The implications of being in a happy, committed marriage relationship are especially significant, as one research study found:

> [The researchers] delved into the question of causality—whether being in a marriage leads to better mental health or if individuals with better mental health are more likely to get married....The direction of causality leans more significantly from the quality and presence of romantic relationships towards improved mental health outcomes. This suggests that being in a committed relationship, such as marriage, tends to enhance one's mental health more profoundly than less committed forms of cohabitation.... The implications of this research are profound, suggesting that interventions aimed at enhancing relationship quality could be as effective as those targeting individual mental health issues.[8]

God created us to love and be loved. How we love—not just how we "live"—really, really matters.

As humbling as it felt at the time, God honored me that day by giving me the most important revelation I've ever received concerning health and wellness. I now make it my purpose to share it with others for the rest of my life. In this book we will discover

- the main features of the love walk, as it is lived out practically in our behavior;
- the biblical basis for making love the central motivation and characteristic of our lives;
- why a pessimistic outlook robs so many believers of their joy and peace—and how to become a faith-filled optimist by choice;
- the key role forgiveness plays in turbo-charging our health;
- and much more!

Join me on the journey of discovering the true source of health and life. I'm sure your own life will be transformed too.

PRAYER AND DECLARATIONS

Lord, I open my heart right now to hear Your message to me through this book. I incline my ear, my heart, and my mind to learn more about the love walk. I want to be as healthy as You made me to be in my body, mind, and emotions. Give me insights into my own life and habits; show me things to change and improve. I commit to obey and implement any fixes or wholesale transformations You bring to my attention. Thank You! Amen.

I am determined to grow in love for the rest of my life.

I will learn things I've never learned before in reading this book.

I will humbly listen to the voice of the Spirit as I take this journey toward a greater expression and experience of love in my life.

CHAPTER 2

TRIUMPH OVER ABUSE AND HOMELESSNESS: MY WIFE'S JOURNEY

MY WIFE, MARY'S, story of forgiveness and tenacity in staying on the love walk is one of the most uplifting and mind-blowing testimonies I've ever heard—and I've heard plenty of them.

Mary was the middle child of nine and spent most of her adolescent years in Florida. When she was in fifth grade, her father went to Vietnam to serve two tours in the US military, but when he returned two years later, he was not the same man. Anger and alcohol had taken over his personality, and their home was soon racked with violence. He actually broke the arm of one of Mary's older brothers one time, and he beat their mother. Gone was the jolly, easygoing dad they had known. In his place was someone tormented by what he had experienced in war.

In some ways Mary's father led a laudable life. Gifted with great intelligence, he came up with the idea to put a whistle and a light on every life vest because while he worked on a US

Navy carrier, he too often saw the jets from the fighter planes blow sailors into the water where they were lost forever. So he helped the navy patent the idea to put a light and a whistle on every life jacket so rescuers could see or hear the men who had gone overboard. That idea became a normal part of the maritime industry, and today vests equipped with lights and whistles are ubiquitous on cruise ships and airplanes. He also helped train astronauts who walked on the moon, and helped design the heat-diffusing tiles on the space shuttle.

At church, Mary's father was a deacon and a well-respected member of the congregation. But at home his dark side came out more and more. The police were called regularly because of his angry raging.

When Mary was in seventh grade, she heard the door to her bedroom open one night while the rest of the house was asleep. Her father came in and tried to assault her sexually. When Mary resisted, he grew violent, and she was terrified but managed to resist him. The next night and every night thereafter, she locked the bedroom door and placed furniture in front of it to keep him from entering. Her mother sometimes intervened and suffered many blows keeping her husband out of Mary's room. One time he knocked a tooth out, and a number of times her blood spattered on the wall. Mary had to clean it up quickly if the police were on their way.

"Please don't say anything to the officers," Mary's mom begged her when the sirens drew near. "They will put your dad in jail, and we will lose all the benefits of the military. How will I feed all these kids?"

Mary came to feel like the sacrificial lamb who suffered so all the other kids could eat. Every night the nightmare repeated itself, and she wondered, "Is this going to be the night my father rapes me?" Every night she fought him off, sometimes with the help of her mother.

Mary continued to grow into an attractive young woman. She joined the cheerleading squad and was one of the popular girls at school. Many guys wanted to date her, but she refused them all. The more she developed physically, the more fearful she became of being assaulted by her father. She took a butcher knife from the kitchen and slept with it next to her bed, thinking, "If he comes in, I'm going to put this right through his chest." He never was able to rape Mary, but the bitterness and hatred she held toward him was immense. She could not stand to be in the same room with him, and she stayed away from the house as much as she could. His actions affected her view of all men and dating. After five years of sometimes nightly attempted assaults, she graduated high school and left the house—for good, she hoped.

An Encounter with Jesus

Mary soon got a job working in a community college. It paid well enough for her to get her own apartment, furnish it, and buy a car. Then a friend invited her to the Assemblies of God church he attended. Having been raised in the Baptist church, Mary knew about the Bible and had gotten saved in the first grade. But she also had witnessed the hypocrisy of religion because of her dad's double life. Not eager to attend church, especially a Pentecostal church with which she was not at all familiar, she only agreed to go because the young man kept pressing her about it.

The preacher that night shared his testimony and gave a sermon on Matthew 6, which says, "If you forgive those who sin against you, your heavenly Father will forgive you. But if you refuse to forgive others, your Father will not forgive your sins" (vv. 14–15, NLT). Mary couldn't believe Jesus had said those words, so she leaned over and asked her friend to show it to her in the Bible. There it was in red; there was no denying it. Mary knew she needed forgiveness like everyone else, but she couldn't countenance the idea of forgiving her father and letting him off the hook so easily. "This is such a raw deal!" she thought. But then she had an idea: "I'm going to go to the altar and talk to God about this and work something out." She thought she could negotiate with God about her situation and persuade Him to give her a pass on forgiving. She was as sincere and confident as she could be as she went forward when the invitation was given.

At the altar, tears flowed as Mary set her case before the Lord. "I know You don't really require this of me," she told Him. "You saw everything I suffered. You don't really mean I need to forgive him." Suddenly the presence of Jesus appeared before her. She did not see Him with her physical eyes, but she knew He was there—and He was weeping over her.

"Why are You crying?" she asked. "I'm the one who went through this nightmare."

"Mary," Jesus said, "if I could make an exemption for anyone right now, you would be that person. But if I did, then I would not be what the Word says I am, for I cannot change."

In that moment Mary had a revelation and a complete understanding that she needed Jesus to be everything the Word says He is, and that this was far more important than her need to hold on to any pain and hatred in her heart.

"Let it go," Jesus said. "Give Me all your hurt and pain, all the betrayal. I rightfully died for it."

Mary sobbed at the altar, letting the tears and pain pour out.

In her heart she heard these words: "Don't let one of those tears go back into your mouth, for I am taking away your bitterness, for oil and vinegar cannot mix. Now, receive My oil."

On the top of her head Mary felt a sensation of hot oil come upon her and flow over her body. She began speaking in tongues and crying, keeping the tears out of her mouth as Jesus had told her to do. In that moment of exchange Mary surrendered all her bitterness and received the most glorious new life in return. As she put it, "I gave Him all my junk, and He gave me all His promises. What a deal!" But still the drama of her young years was far from over.

When Mary got up from the altar some hours later, she felt so light inside it was as if her feet never touched the floor. After virtually floating to the parking lot, she sat in her car and had a thought: She wanted to go see her dad and tell him she forgave him. All hatred had left her body and soul, replaced by excitement, joy, consuming love, and the presence of the Holy Spirit. She pointed her car in the direction of her childhood home.

Both her parents were sitting in the living room when Mary walked in. She went right up to her dad, knelt down, and said, "Dad, I want you to know I forgive you for everything, and I love you." She had never hugged or kissed him before, but she was so full of love that she did just that. With no warning he started shaking and sobbing, his whole body racked with emotion. His shaking went on for so long that Mary's mom became alarmed.

"What have you done to him?" she demanded.

"Nothing! I just told him I forgive him," Mary said.

After watching her husband shake continuously for two hours, Mary's mom called an ambulance to come take him to the hospital. There, the doctors asked him what was happening, and he told them the truth about what he had done to Mary. They admitted him to the psychiatric ward to undergo therapy for what they deemed a mental breakdown.

He spent three months in the hospital, and then one day Mary received a call from her mother telling her the psychiatrist wanted to speak with her. Mary went to the hospital and sat down with the man. He was ready to analyze her, thinking he would be meeting a messed-up girl that day. But when he observed her appearance and began dialoguing with her, he leaned back and said, "I don't understand. How can you be so together after everything I've heard happened to you?"

Mary smiled and replied, "I met Jesus, and He filled me with His love and made everything right."

The psychiatrist shook his head, got up, and said, "Young lady, this is amazing. I've never heard of something like this before, but you're OK."

LOSING A JOB—AND HER HOME

Mary was more than OK; she was on fire for the gospel. She had started a Bible study group at the Assemblies of God church, and it boomed in numbers. She preached to everyone, including people at her job, telling them, "Jesus loves you and has a plan for you." But her boss, a nominal Christian, was annoyed by her constant evangelism and eventually fired her. Unbowed, Mary interviewed for other jobs, certain she would land one quickly to replace the not-insubstantial income she had been earning. In job interviews, when they asked why she was fired from her previous job, she told them the truth, thinking they would be on her side. Results would prove otherwise.

Weeks went by, and Mary still didn't have a job. Before long she couldn't make her car payments or even pay rent. One day she got an eviction notice. The most terrifying possibility to her was the prospect of going back to live with her mother and father.

"God, I'm serving You and teaching Your Word, yet everything is caving in around me," she prayed. "I have nowhere to go, and I have to get this stuff out of my apartment."

Mary's father offered to help her move her items to temporary storage and helped her load it all into a moving truck. He had experienced some changes since his time in the psych ward, and he did not seem so angry anymore. As they were driving down the highway, trucks and cars kept honking at them. He finally looked back to see that the door of the moving truck had not been latched and all of Mary's goods were flying out onto the highway. They pulled over only to witness everything Mary owned be run over and smashed by semitrucks—including her favorite red velvet chair. Her dad started crying.

"Mary, I'm so sorry," he said.

"Dad, it's OK. I don't know what God is doing, but it's OK," she told him.

Stripped of her possessions, her apartment, and her independence, all Mary had left was her car and her church. Worse, she felt paralyzing fear at having to sleep on the couch in the living room of her old home with no door to lock, no furniture to hide behind, no way to protect herself if her father tried to assault her. But night after night, he did not—and he never tried again.

One morning Mary awakened to see her car missing in front of the house. She called the police, and they told her it had been repossessed. That was the point when her mother suffered what might be called a mini–mental breakdown. Thinking that Mary's ongoing presence would cause her husband to start assaulting her again and destroy the life they had rebuilt, she took Mary's few remaining items, threw them into the yard, and said, "Get out of here now. You're not staying here anymore. Take everything that's yours and get out."

Mary gathered her possessions in her arms and walked three and a half miles to the church. She didn't know where else to go or who else to turn to but God. The church, which sat at the end of a cul-de-sac, was empty but unlocked. The second floor had been turned into a room dedicated to prayer, and it had big couches. Mary went up there, plopped down, and began to pray.

"God, what do I do?" she cried out. "Where do I go? Who do I call?"

Exhausted, she lay down on the couch and fell asleep. When she woke up it was past midnight and all the church lights were off. Nobody was there but her.

"OK," she decided, "I'm just going to stay here."

Mary hid her possessions behind the couch and lived in the upper room of that church for more than three months. The caretaker was an older man who did not like to climb the stairs to the second story when he locked up each night. Nobody ever checked if the back door was locked. The pastor's office had a shower Mary used, and she kept an eye on her parents' house to see when they were gone. When they were, she let herself in, got food from the fridge and pantry, and left. She was homeless, and nobody knew about it.

The intimacy she developed with God during those months was life-defining and more valuable than anything else in the world. She read the Word day and night, soaked in God's presence, and sought His face. One day she found the promise in Psalm 27:10: "When my father and my mother forsake me, then the LORD will take care of me." Later, she sensed the Holy Spirit speaking Mark 10:29 to her heart: "There is no one who has left house or brothers or sisters or father or mother or wife or children or lands, for My sake and the gospel's." Because of the sacrifice she was going to have to make, which is far more than I can cover in one chapter, Mary held on to the promise of Psalm 27:10, and today the Holy Spirit has done far more than what He promised He would do.

In that lowest period of her life, Mary became one with her heavenly Father, and it shaped her forever afterward. She also enjoyed His supernatural provision. Friends would invite her to lunch or dinner out of the blue, not knowing she was sometimes going days without food. To keep up the appearance that she was living at home, she asked friends to pick her up at a local gas station on their way to Friday night youth group.

Angelic Visitor

One night, Mary and a friend arrived early for the seven o'clock meeting and ascended the stairs to the upper room where nobody knew Mary was living. There on a couch sat a dark-haired young man they had never seen before. His unexpected presence made them both gasp.

"Hi," he said. "Is this where the Bible study is? I heard about it. Is it OK that I'm here?"

"Yes, of course, welcome," Mary said. They were interrupted by other young people coming in before she could learn more about him.

Fifty young people crammed into the room that night, and the new guy sat there for the whole teaching without opening his mouth. Finally, at the end of the meeting, he spoke up and said, "May I say something?"

The leader gave him permission, and he spoke: "Mary, I have

been given a word from the Lord for you," he said. "The hand of the Lord is mighty upon you, and He shall do mighty things through you. Tomorrow He wants you to go to your parents' home, for you will receive a phone call at noon from a young man. When he calls your house, do exactly as he tells you to do, for this is the will of the Lord."

Mary's first thought was, "How did he know I'm not living at my parents' house? Is he a stalker? Uh-oh!"

"OK, thank you," Mary said, but she was freaked out. Everyone else was affirming, but nobody grasped the import of what he had said. When the stranger left, Mary asked a guy named Jim to go get him so she could learn more about him. "Hurry, hurry!" she said. Jim ran down the stairs, then returned white as a sheet.

"Guys, that new guy is gone," he said. "There is no taillight. He's not in the parking lot. I went down the street; there's nobody there."

"Do you think it was an angel?" they all asked.

But Mary thought he was hiding in the church—and that would be a problem. When everyone else left, she turned off the lights as if she were leaving, but now she was alone in the church.

"Oh, God, help me," she prayed, going through the church room by room, looking under every pew and in every closet, convinced he was there somewhere. But he wasn't. She returned to the upper room, locked the door behind her, and sat up all night terrified.

The next day, Mary considered the man's words again and decided to act on them. She walked to her parents' house a little before noon. Her mom was there, and her dad was at work.

"What do you want?" her mother demanded.

"I left something here I need to get," Mary said.

While she was in her room, the phone rang. Her mother answered and then came to Mary.

"There's a guy on the phone asking for you," she said.

It seemed just as the young man had spoken. Mary walked into the kitchen and picked up the receiver.

"Hello?" she said.

"Hi, my name is Richard, and I'm a student at Oral Roberts University," a voice said. "I know this sounds crazy, but I was at a Bible study, and a friend showed me your picture. I kid you not, I got this strong impression to call you and tell you that you need to come to ORU. I'm just the messenger. I'm being obedient, and I hope you know what to do with this."

"Thank you," Mary said. "I appreciate you calling."

She hung up.

"What's going on?" her mother asked.

"I'm going to ORU," Mary said.

"How are you going to do that?" asked her mother.

"I don't know, but that's not my problem," Mary said. "God is going to make a way."

Both Mary's parents were excited she was leaving town. Her dad went to the junkyard and bought a 1963 Pontiac Bonneville that had been in a wreck. The passenger side was caved in from some impact. He gave the car to Mary as a gift, along with a case of oil and a case of transmission fluid.

"Mary, this car's transmission is shot," he explained. "Every hundred miles you have to put transmission fluid in it. It also does not go in reverse, so everywhere you park, make sure you can go forward from there."

Mary was just excited to have a working car with a radio. But it represented a message about her future as well: God had given her a car that could not go in reverse to make sure there was no going back, no becoming mired in regret or past pain. Before she left, the young people she had been ministering to at the church raised money for her, which became the seed money for her future.

IT'S A FACT!

According to the Mayo Clinic, "letting go of grudges and bitterness can make way for improved health and peace of mind." Chief benefits of doing so include healthier relationships, fewer symptoms of depression, lower blood pressure, improved heart health, and improved self-esteem.[1]

As Mary drove the Bonneville away from her parents' home, she heard the Holy Spirit say, "Take that rearview mirror and turn it away. There's no going back. Everything I am going to do with you is good going forward." She talked with Jesus the whole way down the highway, from Jacksonville to Tulsa, and her main request was this: "I want an apartment with a fireplace because in Florida I didn't need one, but I'm going somewhere cold. Can I have a fireplace?"

When she arrived in Tulsa, the student who had called her met her and took her to the apartment office.

"Honey," the apartment manager said, "I have only one apartment left. It has a fireplace. Is that OK?"

"Ma'am, I don't need to see it," Mary said, almost laughing. "That is my apartment."

She lived there for three years, right next to the pool. She immediately got a job in the mail room on campus and enrolled as a part-time student. The paycheck from her job covered her tuition. She also began doing street evangelism with a group of other fired-up students. The first time I saw her, she was holding a bullhorn on a street corner and preaching the gospel. I thought I had never seen a woman so bold in my life. Throughout our married life, Mary has gone to prisons and jails to tell the story of what she suffered, which resonates strongly with so many women who were molested and abused at young ages.

When people ask her, "How are you able to forgive?" Mary says, "I'm not able to. In our own human ability, we can't forgive with the God kind of forgiveness. It takes full surrender and willingness to let God forgive through you. And it is not for the person you are forgiving; it is for your benefit, your health, your mental clarity, to deliver you from the tormentors that have betrayed and hurt you."

I have observed the power of love in Mary's lifelong example. She has walked the love walk and shown that it works in any circumstance. I have never known a more confident, faith-filled, compassionate, and principled person in my life, and I am proud to be her husband.

The good news is that you and I can take the same love walk and experience amazing results, as we will see.

PRAYER AND DECLARATIONS

Lord, I am Your beloved child. Rescue me from whatever torments and traps have afflicted me in my youth or my adult years. Please help me to walk the love walk no matter what has happened. I choose to forgive everyone who has hurt me, disappointed me, used me, rejected me, abandoned me, humiliated me, and betrayed me. Through the new birth, by accepting

Jesus, I have been given the love of God in my heart, which enables me to forgive everyone, including myself. Help me to recover all that was lost, as You promise to do. Guide my journey supernaturally, making even my lowest times highly productive in You. Draw me closer, and help me to place all my trust in You. Amen.

I declare that I need forgiveness, and I need to forgive. I will not withhold forgiveness from anyone but will allow the mercy of God to flow through me toward all people, by His grace.

I will stop looking in the rearview mirror of life and let the past be covered by the redeeming mercy of God. I declare that my future is much greater than my past.

I will believe God in all circumstances, giving thanks even in seasons of loss and betrayal, because God works all things for good for those who love Him and are called according to His purpose (Rom. 8:28).

CHAPTER 3

YOUR PROGNOSIS: TO LIVE AND LOVE FOREVER

M Y WIFE, MARY, discovered her purpose—her Savior—and chose to stay in the love walk with Him. That became the most crucial decision of her life. Walking in love has an eternal quality. It is like living in heaven right now. You and I were made to live forever spiritually, and love is the fuel that powers our eternal life in God. We were never intended to suffer from diseases, depression, anxiety, or any other deadly condition that has afflicted humanity since the fall. These things came upon us when we departed from love, and perfect wellness only returns when we walk in love. It really is that simple.

When Adam and Eve decided to disobey God, death in its many sordid forms entered the world. We were cut off from the love walk and from the river of God's life. The medical industry was born the day perfect communion with God ended, but nothing mankind has done since then has been able to restore the life we lost by stepping away from Him.

Only love can sustain life; only love can restore our lives today in every way.

If we look back at humanity's history, it is easy to see where things went off track. Separated from the immediate presence of the God who is love, the lifespan of men and women shrank drastically from never-ending to around a thousand years, then rapidly decreased to less than one hundred years. This is the perfect picture of how lack of love diminishes life, reducing it to a nub of what God intended it to be.

We must take this lesson personally: Without the presence of love in our lives, everything diminishes. With love, every good thing is enhanced and strengthened. But when men and women rejected love, the whole race soon turned to violence, exploring great depths of evil and filling the earth with such wickedness and pain that God actually regretted creating us! He sent a worldwide flood to wipe this mayhem off the face of the earth, leaving just eight righteous people through whom He would reestablish all of humanity.

GOD SET A LOVE PLAN IN MOTION

From the beginning God has had a love plan. Adam and Eve sinned, which separated them from God and His plan to bring every willing person back into the fullness of His love through the shed blood of His Son, a plan conceived before the foundation of the world. Again, this indicates God's nature—and you can personalize it. He has had a plan to bring *you* back into relationship with Him. He has a plan right now for you to walk in greater health and vitality than ever before, and it begins with you plugging into His love more than you ever have before.

God did this with Abraham, befriending one man out of all the earth and turning him from a wandering pagan into the father of faith. Generations later, God unfolded more of His plan and gave Abraham's descendants the Law, the priesthood, and the sacrifices through Moses, all of which prophesied the priceless blood of the spotless Lamb that would later be spilled for our redemption. Moses' tabernacle, which represented the one in heaven, became the only place on the planet where blood was shed to atone for the sins of the people each year. These sacrifices did not erase those sins but covered them temporarily. Covered sins remain present, just as a stain in the carpet is still there even though you move the couch or rug over it. The Law began our restoration with God but was not meant to complete it.

Inspired prophets foretold the coming of a Messiah who would lead God's people back into eternal love, peace, and joy in the family of God. These prophecies, written hundreds of years before Jesus' birth, were remarkably specific as to the place of His birth, the nature of His ministry, and the facts about His death. There are around three hundred such prophecies, and the chances of them all coming to pass as they did is so improbable as to serve as a mathematical proof that Jesus was the Son of God—the One sent to bring us back into the love walk for which we were made.

When Jesus willingly went to the cross, He offered the perfect sacrifice once and for all, banishing the need for the blood of sheep, goats, and bulls to atone for sin. Hebrews 7:27 says Jesus' blood offers eternal forgiveness and never needs to be shed again. At the moment He died on the cross, the curtain in the temple was supernaturally torn from top to bottom as the presence of God left the place where it had rested for more than a thousand years (Mark 15:38).

Many Bible scholars believe the curtain was sixty feet high, thirty feet wide, and four inches thick and would have taken a team of oxen to tear in two. But this was God's own declaration that His presence was no longer confined to a temple but would reside inside every human heart that welcomed Him. At that same hour, darkness descended and a great earthquake rocked the region. Jesus was buried, and before rising to life again, He seized the keys of death, hell, and the grave, taking captivity captive, disarming evil powers, and ascending to His Father and ours to present His blood as an eternal redemption for all our sins. His resurrection now stands as an invitation to every man, woman, and child to return to the love walk for which we were designed.

You see, unredeemed people are not equipped to walk in love. They are instead creatures of wrath (Eph. 2:3), and the love of God is not in them. But when you were born again and declared Jesus to be the Savior and Lord of your life, you became a new creation, even a new species of being (2 Cor. 5:17). The very life and nature of God came into your spirit, but your mind has to be renewed every day. You are spirit, soul, and body. When you were born again, your spirit was made alive to God, but you still have the same mind and body. That's why we daily need to renew our minds and crucify our "flesh" (not just our bodies but our sinful desires as well), according to Romans 12:2 and Galatians 5:24. God's love began to flow through you as the sap flows from the roots of a tree through the trunk and into the branches. For the first time, you were connected to life Himself. Jesus said, "I am the vine, you are the branches. He who abides in Me, and I in him, bears much fruit [including the fruit of love]" (John 15:5).

I like how one great evangelist of our day put it: "When Jesus Christ becomes Lord in any life, that man or that woman is then a member of God's family, of divine royalty, of God's kingdom or domain, and His seat of authority and action is then headquartered in that person. When God and a human person are reunited, it is not for the purpose of just sitting and communing together about spiritual blessings. God has restored us to the position for which He originally created Adam and Eve. We are justified by faith in Jesus Christ (Rom. 5:1). It is as though we had never sinned. Now we are His ambassadors. Now we are to subdue and replenish the earth. We are to have dominion over it (Gen. 1:28)."[1]

Now that we have life through Jesus, love is supposed to be the force and motivation that directs our thoughts, words, and actions (Col. 1:13). This is not cheap sentiment or fridge-magnet advice; this is the difference between whether life or death prevails in our bodies, minds, and emotions. It has unlimited implications for every aspect of our health—but we must walk in it. "One thing we've got to realize is that the Holy Spirit can be in your heart in the new birth, but if you don't allow the love of God to dominate you, you'll just walk on in carnality and be defeated," Kenneth Hagin wrote.[2]

LOVE GIVES PHYSICAL HEALTH

"Health" is another way of saying things are functioning as God made them to function. Our salvation is not purely a matter of the spirit but affects our entire being. We should not limit what God did for us and what He wants to give us through our reconciliation to Him. He restored all health to us at the cross! Isaiah 53:5 promised that "by His stripes we are healed."

An article titled "Unlocking the Healing Power of Love: The Link Between Love and Physical Health," based on two studies published in peer-reviewed journals, describes how people who were in loving relationships (in the study) had lower levels of the stress hormone cortisol in their bodies than those who were not in relationships. People in loving relationships also had stronger immune systems than those who were single or in unhappy relationships. Love can even help us recover from physical illnesses, as "research has shown that patients who receive love and support from their family and friends have better outcomes than those who do not. In one study, breast cancer patients who had strong social support had a better quality of life and were more likely to survive their cancer, than those who did not have strong social support."[3]

Increased feelings of being loved—and feeling love for others—appear to lead to a decline in depressive symptoms over time. In one study involving older adults, those who felt loved and expressed love for others had statistically significant lower odds of reporting negative emotions (e.g., depression) than those who reported lower levels of love.[4]

Indeed, "belongingness appears to have multiple and strong effects on emotional patterns and on cognitive processes. Lack of attachments is linked to a variety of ill effects on health, adjustment, and well-being....The need to belong is a powerful, fundamental, and extremely pervasive motivation."[5] Putting "feet" to our love in the form of acts of altruism, such as volunteering and informal helping, can also lead to a significant sense of life satisfaction and positive emotions.[6]

IT'S A FACT!

Let your love be demonstrated in word, by action, by attitude, by giving to others in need, by forgiving, and by forgetting wrongs done to you. Practicing love is the key to faith and the key to living in joy. Practicing love is the key to walking in divine health and becoming disease-resistant.

Jesus came healing the sick from all kinds of afflictions. It's ridiculous to believe that Jesus conquered death but not disease; that He is powerful enough to save our souls but not to redeem our minds from depression and anxiety. Even the old covenant promised divine health, saying, "So you shall serve the LORD your God, and He will bless your bread and your water. And I will take sickness away from the midst of you. No one shall suffer miscarriage or be barren in your land; I will fulfill the number of your days" (Exod. 23:25–26).

In establishing a new covenant, would God remove some of the old benefits? No way! Hebrews 8:6 called ours a "better covenant," not a downgraded version. Health and wellness in our entire bodies, minds, and souls are essential aspects of the better covenant. If we walk with Jesus in love, we will live long and healthy lives free of most diseases. It's a promise.

Picture the Holy Spirit living in a broken-down shack without improving the place or making repairs. It's hard to imagine because that is not how He behaves. When we give our lives to Jesus Christ, the Holy Spirit takes up residence in us—and He comes with great ideas for transforming the place. Jesus said in John 14:16–17 (KJV), "And I will pray the Father, and he shall give you another Comforter, that he may abide with you for ever; even the Spirit of truth; whom the world cannot receive, because it seeth him not, neither knoweth him: but ye know him; for he dwelleth with you, and shall be in you." Paul wrote that the Holy Spirit dwells in us and sheds the love of God abroad in our hearts (Rom. 5:5, KJV). This is a wonderful promise.

Let me ask an obvious question: Does God get sick? Of course not. He is far greater and mightier than any demon, principality, or power—and He does not suffer from illnesses, mental problems, or pathologies. So His design for you and me is not to live in a physical and mental house riddled with problems. Just as the tabernacle of Moses was a perfect replica of the one in heaven, so God intends to adorn our lives with strength and vivaciousness. He is in the business of making everything new and taking pleasure in the renovation. "For we are the temple of the living God; even as God said, I will dwell in and with and among them and will walk in and with and among them, and I will be their God, and they shall be My people" (2 Cor. 6:16, AMPC).

IT'S A FACT!

Agape love is the main sign that you are born again. It is a biblical fact from 1 John 3:14 that we know we have passed from spiritual death into eternal life "because we love the brethren." Love is not a feeling; love is a person. God is love, and love is a commandment, not a suggestion or recommendation.

I have discovered after practicing medicine for more than forty years that we as doctors have missed the most powerful keys to healing and living a long, healthy, and prosperous life full of joy and peace. It is simply following the love commandment and keeping our joy full (John 15:11).

[Love] does not rejoice at injustice and unrighteousness, but rejoices when right and truth prevail.

—1 CORINTHIANS 13:6, AMPC

Some people can better picture what love looks like and feels like because of their upbringing. Some childhoods are saturated with love on all sides—from parents, siblings, grand-parents, friends, cousins, and so on. Other kids grow up in more difficult circumstances and later may have a tougher time defining and even relating to love. But even if we grew up in the most loving home imaginable, God's love is still immeasurably greater. His otherworldly love had never been experienced by mankind (except Adam and Eve) until God sent Jesus. Even the strong love of a mother for her child or a husband for his wife can't match the quality of God's love for us. Paul described divine love this way in a well-known chapter of the Bible:

> Love endures long and is patient and kind; love never is envious nor boils over with jealousy, is not boastful or vainglorious, does not display itself haughtily. It is not conceited (arrogant and inflated with pride); it is not rude (unmannerly) and does not act unbecomingly. Love (God's love in us) does not insist on its own rights or its own way, for it is not self-seeking; it is not touchy or fretful or resentful; it takes no account of the evil done to it [it pays no attention to a suffered wrong]. It does not rejoice at injustice and unrighteousness, but rejoices when right and truth prevail. Love bears up under anything and everything that comes, is ever ready to believe the best of every person, its hopes are fadeless under all circumstances, and it endures everything [without weakening]. Love never fails.
>
> —1 CORINTHIANS 13:4–8, AMPC

The apostle John wrote, "God is love; and he that dwelleth in love dwelleth in God, and God in him. Herein is our love made perfect, that we may have boldness in the day of judgment: because as he is, so are we in this world" (1 John 4:16–17, KJV).

WHERE IS YOUR TREASURE?

From my position in the medical community with an emphasis on treating Christians, I have come to the sad conclusion that most professing Christians believe with their heads but not with their hearts. They have mental belief but not heart belief. Their old man, worldly and carnal, is still on the throne. This explains why they bump along, suffering chronic emotional and physical problems. Their foundation is made of sand. Pastor Keith Moore calls them "the less blessed." They go to church to receive teaching but seldom walk out what they have heard. As born-again children of God they aren't "not blessed," just less blessed.

In light of the majesty and scope of God's health-giving love, let me ask again the question I posed in the introduction: What do you really love? Do you find yourself thinking mostly about pleasures, possessions, and positions? If so, the love of the Father is not in you, according to 1 John 2:15–16. If we are not careful, we may join the ranks of the less blessed Moore talks about. God placed His love inside us when we were born again, and now it is up to us to walk in it. Will we yield to our feelings and behave selfishly, critically, and hatefully? Or will we walk in the selfless love of God that is inside of us? The choice is ours, and it makes all the difference in the world.

Many Christians are spiritual babies and filter most thoughts through the question "How does this benefit me?" Instead we need to ask, "How does this affect my brother or sister?" We need to get out of Me-ville and start loving others with the selfless love of Jesus that is inside us.

Jesus said a wise follower hears His words and puts them into practice, like a man building a house and laying his foundation on the bedrock. Is your love deep enough to rest on the bedrock of Jesus' love? If so, nothing can shake it—that's the very definition of strength. The wind blows, the rain comes down, the river rises and crashes against it, but strong love cannot be shaken by natural occurrences. It overcomes them because the bedrock is unshakable, and we are connected to it.

But if our love sits on the sand and does not touch bedrock, Jesus says we have no strength. We are actually disconnected from the love walk and all the power it offers. When the natural events of life come against us, our lives collapse, proving we were not actually resting on the foundation of Jesus' selfless love. We may have touched it here and there with a selfless act, but our lives are not secure in it. It's like a branch lying near the vine but disconnected from it. The branch will be dead even though it sits so close to that life-giving vine. That describes many Christian lives today: close to the vine, near the bedrock, but not connected to it in such a way as to draw strength from it. So our love is worldly, not divine, and we receive no strengthening joy.

How do we make sure we stay on the love walk, attached to the rock, connected to the vine? Jesus said it plainly: "Keep my commandments" (John 14:15, KJV). Many Christians get worried because they have to keep the Ten Commandments; however, when you love one another, you have fulfilled all the law and the other commandments (Rom. 13:8–10; Gal. 5:14). When people sense strength seeping out of their lives, it's often because they have drifted from obeying God's commandments. Maybe they have a persistent bad attitude, overriding fear, anger, bitterness, or something else. This blotch on their behavior may reside in their blind spot, but the lack of strength indicates something is off.

How about you? If you feel weak, stressed, anxious, or

depressed in mind, body, or emotions, it probably indicates you have departed from the love walk in some area of life. The Bible says, "Be strong in the Lord, and in the power of his might" (Eph. 6:10, KJV). The ultimate answer is to find where that departure is and secure it again to the Person and teachings of Jesus, the rock of our strength. As a doctor, I assure you that the best thing you can do for your health in all areas is to love like Jesus loves—self-lessly, with joy. That's when you become unstoppable. Your confidence and strength are abundant, your joy overflowing. That's the Christian life so many are missing because they only go halfway with God.

If you have begun reading this book and never met Jesus, let's fix that problem right now. Pray this with me, not just from your mind but from your heart:

> *Father, I come to You in the mighty name of Jesus, and I know that You will not turn me away or cast me out, because You said in John 6:37, "The one who comes to Me I will by no means cast out." I believe that Jesus Christ is the Son of God and that He died and was raised from the dead according to the Scriptures. I confess with my mouth that Jesus is Lord of my life, and I believe in my heart that God has raised Him from the dead, and according to Romans 10:9 I am saved. I receive Jesus as both my Savior and the Lord of my life. Your Word says in Romans 10:13, "Whoever calls on the name of the LORD shall be saved," so I am calling on You now, and with confidence I know I am saved and I am Your child! Amen.*

PRAYER AND DECLARATIONS

Now that you are a child of God, you have access to every promise of health and wellness in God's book, the Bible. "No good thing will he withhold from him who loves him," He promised. Jesus said in Luke 11:11–13 (KJV), "If a son shall ask bread of any of you that is a father, will he give him a stone? or if he ask a fish, will he for a fish give him a serpent? Or if he shall ask an egg, will he offer him a scorpion? If ye then, being evil, know how to give good gifts unto your children: how much more shall your heavenly Father give the Holy Spirit to them that ask him?"

Let's claim our inheritance as children of the King! Father, we boldly come before You and ask You to lead us in this journey of full health and restoration—body, mind, and emotions. Say the following out loud:

I declare that You have only good things in mind for me.

Your thoughts and intentions toward me are to give me a hope and a future far better than any I have ever dreamed.

You are well able to redeem and transform every area of my life and my past.

Now, friend, let's embark on this love walk together to discover the vibrant health it brings to all areas of life.

CHAPTER 4

TAKING THE LOVE WALK

ARY AND I both have strong personalities, to put it mildly. When we were young, we often would say unkind things without giving much thought, which did neither of us any good. Nobody gained by these thoughtless interactions, and in fact we sometimes created messes we then had to clean up! Over time, as we gained years and maturity, we made the conscious decision to speak more kindly to one another. Mary and I like to start our mornings by speaking softly to each other—no harsh tones, no harsh words. We know how good it feels to kick things off relationally that way instead of stewing on what was said the night before or choosing to be irritable. Life-giving interactions feed both of us and set our compass in the right direction. As someone wise said, it's nice to be nice.

This might seem overly simple, but choices like that have a much bigger impact than you may suspect. They put us in the river of God's life-giving love, step by step, little by little. In that river, love multiplies the more we give it away through acts of kindness and attitudes of gratitude and gentleness. Worldly, selfish "love" disappears under the abounding water of that river, and our days become saturated with a sense of God's peace and care.

My motivation for walking in love is not only spiritual. In my professional opinion, the healthiest patients I have are the ones who consistently walk in peace and joy and stay in the rushing current of God's love. These people generally have better cardiovascular health, their blood pressure is generally much lower, they are more resistant to heart disease and cancer, their immune systems usually function better, and they almost always live to a ripe old age in good health.

Dr. Helen Riess, an associate clinical professor of psychiatry at Harvard Medical School, has noted that love combats loneliness, a condition that "stimulates anxiety, which is mediated by different neurotransmitters, like norepinephrine. Also, cortisol and adrenaline levels rise when people feel insecure and threatened." Being in love and feeling close to another person can lessen anxiety and anxiety's poor health effects, she says.[1]

Other studies confirm this, pointing to the same culprit— elevated cortisol—which can result from loneliness-induced stress. Our bodies interpret this condition as danger, and when the stress continues over days and weeks, it can dysregulate our cardiovascular and immune systems and our metabolism. All this contributes to heart disease, diabetes, cancer, and other debilitating health issues, according to a study that examined the impact of social connections on mortality risk.[2] Chronic inflammation is also caused by a "systemic release of blood proteins that prep the immune system to deal with danger or injury," reads one article. "As with cortisol, loneliness-related stress can cause inflammation to become chronic, says Dr. Robert Waldinger, director of Harvard University's Adult Development Survey. And as with elevated cortisol, that can lead to a host of diseases."[3]

Love and togetherness also keep us healthier because, among

other things, close friends and spouses make us go to the doctor and pay attention to warning signs we might be inclined to ignore. "There's a lot of denial around medical illness, and individuals are more likely to shrug off something and say, 'This can't be serious,'" Riess told *Time* magazine.[4] Data shows that people in loving relationships benefit from the people close to them noticing things like suspicious moles, unusual or worrisome changes in habits, and abnormal bruising, which can be a sign of conditions such as leukemia, kidney disease, and Cushing's disease, Riess said.[5]

Loving people enjoy long, healthy lives because they are walking in life itself. This same reality is available to each one of us.

The New Testament Greek language uses the word *zoe* to describe the "God kind" of life. It is the life we begin to partake of when we receive Jesus as our Lord and Savior. It is synonymous with His love, and as we walk in the love of God, the fleshly nature is transformed by the renewing of our minds in God's Word, especially scriptures on love (Rom. 12:2). *Zoe* is eternal, everlasting life, the nature and love of God. But this *zoe* life is not in our minds or our bodies; it is in our spirit man. Receiving God's love is the greatest miracle any person can experience because God is imparting His very nature and being into our human spirits. As the apostle Peter put it,

> His divine power has given to us all things that pertain to life and godliness, through the knowledge of Him who called us by glory and virtue, by which have been given to us exceedingly great and precious promises, that through these you may be partakers of the *divine nature*, having escaped the corruption that is in the world through lust.
> —2 PETER 1:3–4, EMPHASIS ADDED

Paul also underlined this truth in 2 Corinthians 5:17, saying, "Therefore if any man be in Christ, he is a new creature [new species of being]: old things are passed away; behold, all things are become new" (KJV). God's love transforms us from one type of creature to another! His love enlivens everything it touches, which is why it is the critical ingredient in our physical and mental health as well.

Once you are aware of it, this life-giving flow of God's love shows up everywhere in the New Testament. Jesus said in John 10:10, "I am come that they might have life [zoe], and that they might have it more abundantly" (KJV).

John wrote of Jesus, "In him was life [zoe]; and the life [zoe] was the light of men" (1:4, KJV). Jesus said in John 6:63, "It is the Spirit who gives life [zoe]; the flesh profits nothing. The words that I speak to you are spirit, and they are life [zoe]."

Jesus said, "For as the Father hath life in himself; so hath he given to the Son to have life in himself" (John 5:26, KJV).

Even the most famous verse in the Bible highlights the life-giving love of God: "For God so loved the world, that he gave his only begotten Son, that whosoever believeth in him should not perish, but have everlasting life [zoe]" (John 3:16, KJV).

Paul wrote in Romans 6:23, "For the wages of sin is death, but the gift of God is eternal life [zoe] in Christ Jesus our Lord."

John wrote at the end of his Gospel, "these are written that you may believe that Jesus is the Christ, the Son of God, and that believing you may have life [zoe] in His name" (John 20:31).

The love of God and the life of God are one and the same—and this reality flows to us from the very dwelling place of God. This zoe life and the agape love of God are relayed as we crucify our flesh daily, renew our minds daily, and walk in the revelation of Galatians 2:20, "I have been crucified with Christ; it is no longer I who live, but Christ lives in me." We then must allow Jesus to live through us.

A River from the Throne

The Bible often speaks of the life of God in terms of water. There is a reason for that, and it has to do with the very origins of this headwaters of health.

In the Book of Revelation, John witnesses the life of God, which is another way of saying the love of God, flowing from His throne in massive volumes, running like a river down the center of the heavenly city, the New Jerusalem. "Then the angel showed me a river with the water of life, clear as crystal, flowing from the throne of God and of the Lamb. It flowed down the center of the main street" (Rev. 22:1–2, NLT).

Elsewhere in Revelation, John wrote, "For the Lamb on the throne will be their Shepherd. He will lead them to springs of life-giving water. And God will wipe every tear from their eyes" (7:17, NLT).

The love and *zoe* life of God literally billows from the throne of God in unending supply. It courses through the city of the great King, feeding all its springs—and then pours into and through each child of God! From there it gushes out to the world. This may be a new thought to you or a reality that is worth greater consideration. The term Jesus used describes this living water of God's love as something that leaps up, jumps up, bubbles up, or gushes up.[6] The picture could not be clearer: We were made to be like wide-open fire hydrants or geysers of love that cleanse and enliven us while rushing out to those around us. For this reason, Jesus said the world would know who His followers were by their love for one another (John 13:35).

The love of God is not merely emotional or metaphorical. It

is not an imaginary concept. The river of life-giving love is literal, even though it's supernatural. It affects everything about us from our physical health to our emotions to our worldview to our daily words and actions.

ON THE BANKS OF THE RIVER

The tragedy is that so few Christians live in the constant flow of God's love. The church we see around us has virtually no power, no overflow of love, no joy or peace, hardly anything to show for being God's children. When was the last time you met a believer and said, "Wow! I see the love in that person's eyes. It's like love is gushing out of their entire being!" More to the point, how often have you felt as if unlimited love was flowing out of you?

I see a lot of Christian patients, and I can tell you the Christian population is just as depressed and in a mess as people without Christ. God's love restores, heals, and rejuvenates—but only when we walk in it. For most Christians—and I say "most" with sadness and certainty—the love within them is only a trickle. It is there; it is recognizable and strong enough to save them from hell, but it's only minimally life-changing for them and those around them. Jesus promised us that "He who believes in Me, as the Scripture has said, out of his heart will flow rivers of living water" (John 7:38). With God's love bubbling up inside of us, how can we be so blasé, bland, and "blah" about things? Where is the overflow that changes circumstances and relationships around us?

In Luke 7, Jesus walked around with power literally coming out of Him. All people had to do was touch Him and they were healed! This also happened to Peter, when people were healed as they got close enough to him, and to Paul, when people were healed when they merely touched a piece of cloth that had touched him. The love of God has a presence, a proximity, and if I can put it this way, a substance. It impacts the natural realm. This has every implication for our physical bodies in addition to every other aspect of our beings.

The measure of love flowing out of us is exactly commensurate with how much we are walking and abiding in that river from God's throne. It's like a gauge. You can check your own love level to tell how much you are abiding in Christ. It's a metric you cannot hide. Everyone has a kind of love sensor in their soul that can pretty accurately detect how much love another person is walking in. Maybe we don't see it with complete precision as we do a meter on our car, but we sense it if a person is walking in a lot of love, joy, and peace. We trust that person more. We want to be around them and emulate them in our own behavior. Similarly, we get "bad vibes" from people who walk in selfishness and the ways of their father, the devil.

When we walk in love, the flow washes away our own toxic thoughts, even toxic elements in our bodies. This is because peaceful people are more relaxed, and relaxation allows our bodies to unclench and release metabolic waste material that's trapped in tense, tight, contracted muscles. Just as running water indicates life, and usually no algae, disease, or scum grows there, so the river of love washes away toxins and waste products in our bodies and minds. Paul calls it the "washing of water by the word" (Eph. 5:26). That isn't just picturesque phrasing. It is literal. We are washed by the Word, spiritually and physically. Our health is largely determined by how fully we walk in the river of God's love.

I often wonder how many healings and healing prayers would not be needed if people were abiding in the love of God.

How much of a church's or ministry's time is taken up solving problems people create in their own lives by neglecting to wake up each morning and step into that river of love? A healthy, powerful church abides together in love that is never stagnant and flows out of each member. Love is meant for much more than just healing and transforming our minds and bodies; it is intended to emanate outward from us and revolutionize the entire earth.

I have noticed that preachers and ministers take apart the love walk piece by piece and teach on isolated components of it rather than on love itself. There are messages on "How to Have Peace," "Increasing Your Joy," and "Exercising Your Faith." Those are all aspects of love, so why don't we teach on the main thing, which empowers them all? It makes no sense to separate them from this central reality of the kingdom. At the very least, love should be part of every message a Christian preaches.

IT'S A FACT!

An estimated 7 million US children from ages three to seventeen have been diagnosed with ADHD at some point, according to a 2022 national survey of parents. Boys (15 percent) were more likely to be diagnosed with ADHD than girls (8 percent).[7]

THE NEED TO ABIDE

We live in what is best described as a fast-paced, ADD/ADHD society, with roughly 11 percent of US children having been diagnosed with ADHD at some point, according to a 2022 survey.[8] Everyone seems to possess shortened attention spans compared to people in previous generations. I'm convinced that almost all of us are affected by this trend to some degree. Is it even possible anymore to distinguish between people who genuinely have ADHD and those who do not? Not if you examine most people's habits. People lose focus in church. They lack the mental stamina to go deeply into a topic. Even social media and internet videos are becoming "shorts" and "reels," brief enough to deliver something of seeming value quickly so people can move on to the next. The only way some people can "abide" is by sitting on the couch or in bed for hours scrolling through five hundred posts. Our capacity for soaking in the river of life is ebbing away as our culture speeds up and people become less able to direct their attention to one topic for any length of time.

I remember regularly having three-hour church services with Benny Hinn when he pastored in Orlando, and nobody thought anything of it. I remember tarrying at many altars, waiting on the Lord. As people remained and gave God room to move, amazing things happened. Demons came out of people, believers were baptized in the Holy Spirit, true repentance and reconciliations were achieved, bodies were healed. How many times do people today rush past their miracle, their deliverance, their healing because they don't have the patience and self-control to stay for a while in God's presence?

Daniel 12:4 records that the angel Gabriel prophesied this reality twenty-five hundred years ago when he said, "many shall run to and fro, and knowledge shall increase." These astonishingly prescient words depict a time of unprecedented knowledge, such as we live in today in this Information Age. Futurist R. Buckminster Fuller first identified the "knowledge doubling curve" in his 1981 book *Critical Path*, in which he stated that human knowledge had doubled approximately every century until around 1900, but by the end of World War

II it was doubling every twenty-five years.[9] "Years later, IBM researchers published a report that...predicted that '*by 2020, knowledge would double every 12 hours,* fueled by the Internet of Things.'"[10]

But this explosion of knowledge is coupled with a restlessness that keeps us chasing satisfaction all across the globe while never finding it. This must be why many preachers don't instruct their people to abide in God's love but rather teach to the shortened attention spans of our culture. The most they hope to accomplish is to help their hearers get along in the broken-down lives they lead—equipping them for ongoing failure and shallowness on their way to heaven. Meat never gets served, only milkshakes and gospel lattes. I've seen people who have attended church regularly for fifty years who are still eating spiritual "baby food"! They should be fathers and mothers in the Lord, but they remain infants because they have not abided in love. They live mostly on the banks of the river of life.

Sadly, I've come to realize that many believers don't even know this river of heavenly love is available to them as a lived reality. They are conscious of a lot of things—their careers, entertainment, health problems, relationships, retirement plans—but not of the ever-available love of God. Some Christians take a sip of that love now and then, but too few of us plunge in headfirst and gulp it in. We desperately need a revelation and ongoing awareness of the power of the love of God if we are to break free of the problems that plague us.

There is no way to live effectively on the banks of the river. We must step into the flow of God's love daily.

BECOMING CONSCIOUS OF GOD'S LOVE

Many church leaders and preachers treat saints like they are sinners, producing a heightened consciousness of sin, failure, weakness, and unworthiness. These things drain the life and health out of us, increasing stress, depression, and anxiety. The gospel is not primarily about reminding us of who we were without Christ but of who we are while abiding in His love. You might not realize it by listening to some popular preachers, but God looks at us when we are born again as though sin had never touched us. He sees us as accepted in the Beloved (Eph. 1:6), robed in His righteousness. In His eyes you and I are "in Christ." He sees His own nature in us.

Second Corinthians 5:21 says, "For He made Him who knew no sin to be sin for us, that we might become the righteousness of God in Him." Ephesians 4:24 says to "put on the new man which was created according to God, in true righteousness and holiness." Hebrews 4:16 exhorts us, "Let us then fearlessly and confidently and boldly draw near to the throne of grace (the throne of God's unmerited favor to us sinners), that we may receive mercy [for our failures] and find grace to help in good time for every need [appropriate help and well-timed help, coming just when we need it]" (AMPC). By contrast, so many Christians act as if it says, "Let us come full of fear, timidly, awkwardly, feeling unworthy, and crawling on all fours."

We desperately need to turn our love consciousness way up and our unrighteousness consciousness way down. In no way am I making light of sin or giving excuses for bad behavior, but love has a way of overcoming and erasing those habits and tendencies when we keep our minds firmly attached to the author of love. We need to put before ourselves the astounding revelation Jesus gave in John 15:9–10 when He said, "As the

Father loved Me, I also have loved you; abide in My love. If you keep My commandments, you will abide in My love, just as I have kept My Father's commandments and abide in His love." We need to marinate in the truth that "God would make known what is the riches of the glory of this mystery among the Gentiles; which is Christ in you, the hope of glory" (Col. 1:27, KJV).

First John 4:4 similarly assures us, "Little children, you are of God [you belong to Him] and have [already] defeated and overcome them [the agents of the antichrist], because He Who lives in you is greater (mightier) than he who is in the world" (AMPC).

This is the transforming truth of the gospel, and the more we dwell on it and in it, the more we are changed into His likeness.

Of all the Christian men and women I have known and worked with, none was so full of love, joy, and positive energy as T. L. Osborn, the great healing evangelist who lived to be eighty-nine years old before going to be with the Lord. I thank God for TL because to me he was the picture of love. It flowed from his whole being and countenance. He seemed to walk with God uniquely and powerfully. I have often considered his example and asked myself why more Christians are not like that. The answer, I found, is in one of Osborn's own teaching series, called "Behold the Son." In it he said we have to get the revelation of Christ in us, who is the hope of glory (Col. 1:27). This endows us with supernatural strength to fight the good fight of faith, to believe God's promises and to stand on them, and to walk in love by staying in communion with Christ.

BEHOLD JESUS

I like how Osborn put it: To behold Jesus, we must perceive the plan, receive the Lamb, and believe the Man, Christ Jesus! We fervently hold with a faith unshakable to Christ unchangeable. The Osborns at one point beheld Jesus Himself in a visitation, but not before experiencing failure on the mission field. They sailed for India when TL and Daisy were only twenty and twenty-one years old, and they struggled to spread the gospel. T. L. Osborn writes:

> We were there for nearly one year. We could not convince the Hindus and the Moslems that Jesus Christ was the Son of God, that He is risen from the dead and that He lives today. We did not understand about God's miracle-working power. We had no way to prove to them the current evidence of God's love. It was written in the Bible, but we could not give them living proof that the Bible is God's word.[11]
>
> One day, we heard a woman preach at a great camp meeting. Her subject was, "If You Ever See Jesus, You Will Never Be the Same Again." The next morning at 6 o'clock, Jesus Christ came into our bedroom. I saw Him like I would see anyone that walked into our room. I lay there helpless in His presence. I could not move a finger or a toe. Water poured from my eyes, yet I was not conscious of weeping. I learned that the human body cannot stand the presence of Jesus.
>
> After a long while, I was able to move myself and I lay on the floor, face down. That afternoon, when I walked out of that room, I knew I was a new man. I knew I was not proclaiming a dead religion. I was proclaiming a living Jesus. I knew that this world wanted to know that He is really alive. From that day, the fire of our desire

> burned brighter. We had a lot more perspiring to do, but
> we knew that we had found the secret to convincing the
> non-Christian masses that Jesus Christ is the same today
> as He ever was.[12]

Not everyone experiences a visitation from Jesus, but TL taught that every person can get a revelation of who is inside us. We saw earlier that we are the temple of the living God, His precious children, His chosen people in whom He lives and manifests His ways and nature. We have to embrace the vision of who is living inside us—the resurrected, glorified Christ, not Christ on the cross. It is the glorified Jesus of Revelation 1:14–16: "His head and hair were white like wool, as white as snow, and His eyes like a flame of fire; His feet were like fine brass, as if refined in a furnace, and His voice as the sound of many waters; He had in His right hand seven stars, out of His mouth went a sharp two-edged sword, and His countenance was like the sun shining in its strength."

In verse 18 of that passage Jesus describes Himself as "He who lives, and was dead, and behold, I am alive forevermore. Amen. And I have the keys of Hades and of Death." Wow! This doesn't just mean He is alive and conscious but that He is at peak health all the time—and this man lives in us by His Spirit. Jesus said in the Gospels that God is the God of the living, not the dead (Mark 12:27). That includes you and me. Jesus glows with health, and His children can be as full of life as He is. His health is ours because we are one spirit with Him (1 Cor. 6:17).

In nature, God gave a living symbol of our need to bask in Him by the fact that our bodies crave sunlight. Our skin drinks it in, and it causes our bodies to produce vitamin D. God made sunlight beneficial because it is in our nature and design to behold the Son Himself. This is why Paul said to fix our eyes on things that are unseen (2 Cor. 4:18). John testified that he and the other apostles beheld and touched Him who is eternal life (1 John 1:1). Our God is not distant and ethereal but dwells in our bodies.

While shame and other negative feelings cause emotional, mental, and physical disease and eventually death to abound in our bodies, the cure is so simple that we often overlook it: gaze upon the eternal Light of Christ, for "They looked to Him and were radiant, and their faces were not ashamed" (Ps. 34:5). As John the Baptist declared, "Behold! The Lamb of God" (John 1:29). A healthy lifestyle starts with beholding Jesus, considering who He is, reading about Him in the Word. Our looking literally determines our quality and quantity of living.

Osborn says, "Your greatest personal development is to get God's view of the world, to see people as God sees them, to absorb His nature and to get in harmony with His emotions until He lives and loves and lifts people through you."[13]

Radiant with Health

When Psalm 34 says those who look to God are "radiant," it means health emanates from their bodies. They have robust circulatory systems, rosy cheeks, a glowing face, bright eyes, and a great complexion. Reading the Word of God brings health by its nature. It's like taking nutrients and vitamins; it is true bread. Yes, we still need natural food and supplements, but the Word of God has a physical effect on our bodies. It is not just spiritual food; it is literal health to our bones.

As part of my health routine, I listen to some key sermons over and over, dozens of times, because every time I do they impart something new to me. Mary sometimes asks me, "Why are you listening to this same sermon over and over again?" It's because my mind, body, and spirit vibrate to the revelation in these messages. Through them I am beholding the Son in a fresh way.

IT'S A FACT!

The average attention span of a human is 8.25 seconds and decreased by almost 25 percent from 2000 to 2015. Attention spans can range from two seconds to over twenty minutes. Women usually have longer attention spans than men. Almost one in ten people forget their own birthday from time to time.[14]

The main way we behold the Son is to consider Jesus' example in the Bible in light of our circumstances. When you feel overwhelmed by guilt over past sin, behold Jesus on the cross where He vanquished the record of your sins—they don't exist to God anymore! When you doubt that God can work in your difficult situation, behold Jesus going through the villages performing miracles. Never did He doubt that blind eyes would open or deaf ears would hear. He never failed to heal, and He will not fail in your life if you submit things to Him.

Osborn said in one of his great messages that people all over the world pray for a miracle of healing, not understanding the redemptive power of the gospel to heal. We don't need a miracle, he said—we just need the gospel! Osborn observed that Western churches don't see as many healings as churches in other parts of the world because people have been preprogrammed to think they are suffering for Christ when they are sick. They bear up under the afflictions they believe God gave to them.

It seems that before Americans can get healed, they need

someone to preach out of them all that's been preached into them about the subject of healing! We make God inadequate and cruel when He is neither. Within the gospel is all the power we need to be physically and mentally healed of any affliction or disease. The God of miracles in India and Africa is the same God we serve in America—but we must walk in the river of God's love by faith to receive all the benefits of the gospel.

When health or emotional problems come upon you, do as TL recommended and quit chasing your anxieties down each rabbit trail. Instead, behold the Son! Behold Him through the gospel, because it is a gospel that cannot be changed. If you believe that by His stripes we are healed, you will be well. No disease can stand in the face of that prophetic utterance. If Jesus took our diseases, then we no longer have them. We no longer own them. A transaction has been made. He suffered our diseases. They have done their worst. Their power is gone.

You may travel to revival services or healing crusades or conventions. You might fast for healing. But none of this augments the gospel one bit. The power of healing is there the whole time. It just must be beheld. Jesus said, "I have come," and He has never left (John 10:10). His health is yours and mine to grab hold of. We do this by agreeing with the prophets who foretold it. We believe with the Word of God that proclaims it. We come into alignment with the Christ who embodies it and never changes. We stand in the healing stream of the eternal, prophetic message of the gospel—the river of God's love.

MY DINNER WITH BENNY HINN

Benny Hinn has been my pastor and good friend for more than forty years. Recently Mary and I had dinner with Benny at his condo in Florida, where he told us about a huge crusade in Africa he had just been a part of. At the crusade he met with some pastors who were worried because about one-third of them had lost their churches due to an onslaught of online criticism from fellow pastors. One pastor asked Benny what the pastors should do to prevent or curtail this onslaught of online attacks from other pastors that were destroying their ministries and causing many churches to close.

Benny prayed silently and immediately received the answer by the Holy Spirit. Benny answered that as long as the pastors are crucified with Christ, then it is not them (the pastors) the others are attacking but Christ who lives in them—and Christ Jesus will fight their battles for them. He has been doing that very thing for almost fifty years of ministry, Benny said, and even though at times it appeared his ministry would go under due to attacks from others, including the national news media, Jesus always came through for him. When he was attacked, he simply confessed out loud that he had been crucified with Christ and it was not Benny who was running the ministry but Jesus because Benny's life had been crucified with Christ. Christ then fought Benny's battles, and he never went under but was always victorious—because he is crucified with Christ.

That revelation was imparted to Mary and me when we heard this testimony, so every day we now confess that we are crucified with Christ and it is no longer we that live but Christ who lives in us. In Colossians 1:26–27 Paul calls it "the mystery which was hidden [from angels and mankind] for ages and generations, but has now been revealed to His saints (God's people). God [in His eternal plan] chose to make known to them how great for the Gentiles are the riches of the glory of this mystery, which is Christ in and among you, the hope and guarantee of [realizing the] glory" (AMP). Christ living in you is the key and the mystery—being crucified with Christ, dying to ourselves and living to Jesus.

Galatians 2:20 (AMP) is the key scripture:

> I have been crucified with Christ [that is, in Him I have shared His crucifixion]; it is no longer I who live, but Christ lives in me. The life I now live in the body I live by faith [by adhering to, relying on, and completely trusting] in the Son of God, who loved me and gave Himself up for me.

Most Christians are not crucified with Christ. Their flesh is still on the throne. We must grasp this reality and live in it. Romans 6:6 tells us, "We know that our old self [our human nature without the Holy Spirit] was nailed to the cross with Him, in order that our body of sin might be done away with, so that we would no longer be slaves to sin" (AMP).

Did you catch that? Our sinful nature was nailed to the cross along with Jesus, and we must see and believe that to walk the love walk.

Second Corinthians 6:16 (AMPC) asks,

> What agreement [can there be between] a temple of God and idols? For we are the temple of the living God; even as God said, I will dwell in and with and among them and will walk in and with and among them, and I will be their God, and they shall be My people.

This is so powerful—God is living in us, with us, and among us. God is love! So 1 John 4:16 tells us, "We have come to know [by personal observation and experience], and have believed [with deep, consistent faith] the love which God has for us. God is love, and the one who abides in love abides in God, and God abides continually in him" (AMP). And Romans 13:10 says, "Love does no wrong to a neighbor [it never hurts anyone]. Therefore [unselfish] love is the fulfillment of the Law" (AMP).

God is love and He dwells in us, and we in Him. He fights our battles for us. Our job is to stay crucified and stay in the love walk. The last thing Jesus prayed before being crucified was "that they all may be one; just as You, Father, are in Me and I in You, that they also may be one in Us, so that the world may believe [without any doubt] that You sent Me" (John 17:21, AMP).

Amazing! By our love, people will know we belong to God. The Word of God says that in the last days people will hate and betray one another (Matt. 24:10). This is happening in the church too, and the backbiting and strife is affecting ministries and tearing churches apart. We should instead be walking in love. We should be known by our good fruit, not the negative fruit so many Christians are bearing. When we are crucified with Christ, we produce beautiful fruit, and that is the key to the Christian lifestyle. God is love. As we love one another, He works on our behalf and we produce "love fruit," the most beautiful fruit there is.

Prayer and Declarations

Here are some simple declarations you can speak to yourself, as I do, throughout each day to keep the love and *zoe* life of God before me:

> *I have the life and nature of God in me according to John 1:4, "In Him was life, and the life was the light of men."*

I am a new creature, and the zoe *life and nature of God are part of my spirit man. "Old things have passed away; behold, all things have become new" (2 Cor. 5:17).*

The love of God has been shed abroad in my heart by the Holy Spirit, according to Romans 5:5. His love was freely given to me in the new birth, and I allow it to flow out of me and touch everyone I encounter.

"I am crucified with Christ: nevertheless I live; yet not I, but Christ liveth in me" (Gal. 2:20, KJV). The love of God is released as I stay crucified with Christ.

The God of life and love lives and walks in me, and His love shines out of me (Matt. 5:16).

God has generously shined the light of His love in every formerly dark place in my life (Isa. 43:19).

God's love flows from me like a river (John 7:38)!

Father God, teach me to walk in the river of Your love, which flows from the very center of existence, Your great throne. Help me to choose love daily, moment by moment, and to feel the strength of Your joy and peace. I behold Your Son in all His glorious radiance, and I set my mind on things pertaining to resurrection life, not death. My problems are pip-squeaks in light of the almighty power of God. Thank You for welcoming me into the depths of that river of love, and help me to let it flow to a hurting, love-starved world. Amen!

CHAPTER 5

LOVE IN ACTION

MY MOM WAS the most beautiful woman most people had ever met, and she was also a great woman of God who walked in the joy of the Lord. When she went to be with the Lord at age eighty-seven, it occasioned one of the most remarkable supernatural events in Mary's and my life.

Mom, whose name was Kitty, was one in a million in terms of beauty. People would walk up to her in public when she was younger and tell her she looked like a movie star, and they were right. When she entered a room or a grocery store, people stared at her. She was perfectly put together, blonde, and porcelain-skinned. In the sun, her hair glistened like spun gold.

When my then-girlfriend, Mary, first laid eyes on her, Mary wilted and said, "Gee, Don, you didn't warn me your mom was this pretty! This is the standard I have to live up to?" Mom just laughed and hugged Mary. Mom was beautiful inside and out. She walked in the love of the Lord like few people I have known.

Before my father died, Dad and Mom sold their store. Then Dad's brother, Thomas, gave Mom a job at the bank he owned. It was a generous act, and it also probably extended her life. She served as a switchboard operator, which kept her brain working and gave her somewhere to be and people to socialize with. People were drawn to her because she was so full of joy. Everyone loved Kitty. But for whatever reason, though Mom was deeply grateful for that job, she never thanked Thomas and his wife, Ann, for giving it to her.

After many years, Mom suffered a major stroke and slipped into a coma for a few days. During this time, Mary had a dream at three o'clock one morning. In it, my mom came to her looking young and vivacious, as she did when Mary had first met her. Light beamed from Mom's face, and in the dream Mary was so overcome by her beauty, her youthful, strong voice, and the love radiating from her that she began to cry. Then my mom spoke.

"Mary, please go to Ann and Thomas for me," she said. "I need you to go and check on them."

As my mom continued to speak, Mary in the dream cried so hard she had trouble deciphering all the words. She woke up sobbing, feeling that she had been with my mother in the presence of God. She got out of bed, went into the living room, and waited for me to wake up. When I did, Mary made an announcement.

"Don, your mom's gone," she said.

"No, no," I said.

I kept believing that Mom would wake up.

"No, she's gone," Mary repeated. "She came to me in a dream and wants me to call Ann and Thomas, but I was so overwhelmed by how young and full of life she looked, and by the strength of her voice, that I missed the last few words of what she said."

I believed what Mary told me, though none of us were

expecting Mom to go home so soon. Within an hour my brother, Dan, called.

"Mom's gone," he said.

Mary had been right—and now she had a task to perform. But before calling Thomas and Ann, she needed to know what exactly to tell them. Mary prayed, "Lord, what was Kitty saying? Why was she wanting me to call them?"

Thank them, came the response in her heart, and it struck Mary with heavenly force. That was the message she was to convey. She called Thomas and Ann that same day.

"Kitty visited me in the middle of the night, and she has a message for you," Mary told them as they both listened on the phone. "The message is: 'Thank you.'"

Thomas and Ann began weeping, and Mary joined them in their tears. It was exactly what they needed to hear. Mom had appreciated the job at Thomas' bank, but that was not enough. That appreciation needed to be expressed, and it seems God gave her a chance to finally convey that message before she entered heaven.

The chapel in Forest, Mississippi, was packed for the funeral. How many funerals for people in their late eighties draw hundreds of people? My mom's did. It seemed the whole town of Forest turned out to honor her.

I gave the eulogy that day and recounted Mom's visit to Mary in the dream. In front of Ann and Thomas and many of his bank employees who were in attendance, I got to tell about the gratitude Mom had expressed. Thomas was honored, and everyone was so choked up they could barely talk.

"Thank you for giving my mom a job," I ended by saying. It felt profound and so right.

Love always requires action. Thoughts and feelings alone

don't usually count. In my mom's case, she needed to say thanks for a gift she had received. The Bible commands, "In everything give thanks" (1 Thess. 5:18). Notice it doesn't say, "In everything, feel thankful." If we do not give it, it does not count. In similar manner, Psalm 34 says, "I will *bless* the LORD at all times....Oh, *magnify* the LORD with me" (vv. 1, 3, emphasis added). When we express thanks for everything, it opens doors for more—but we must actively give our thanks and bless the Lord, magnify His name, and much more.

PUTTING OUR LOVE TO WORK

God's love always manifests in our behavior. Joshua 1:8 connects meditating on the Word to doing. It reads, "that you may be careful *to do*" (NIV, emphasis added). Likewise, James the brother of Jesus said in James 1:22, "But be ye doers of the word, and not hearers only, deceiving your own selves" (KJV). Later, in James 2:20, he wrote, "faith without works is dead" (KJV). Works means corresponding action.

Love must be exercised. There is no such thing as deedless, wordless love. John wrote in 1 John 3:18, "My little children, let us not love in word or in tongue; but in deed and in truth" (KJV).

I have noticed that possessing knowledge never changes anyone. It is the doing that changes us and others. Just as medical treatments don't work if you merely know about them or think about them, so love doesn't work unless you actively do something to express it.

When I go to the gym to exercise in the afternoons, I see the same guys coming in day after day, sometimes four or five days a week. At first some of them were swimming in their big sweatshirts and workout clothes, sporting tiny little muscles.

But I watched them jump on these machines and work hard to sculpt their bodies the way they wanted. Even though I don't know these guys personally, I have watched their biceps go from maybe ten inches in circumference to sixteen inches or more! Because they do it consistently, they get good results. Nothing would change if they lay around at home dreaming of what they wanted to look like. Going to the gym regularly has made all the difference in the world.

Beholding Jesus, as we looked at earlier, always leads to behaving as Jesus does. When we get a vision of who Jesus is, we also get a vision of who we are and what God wants us to do. First John 3:8 says Jesus was manifested to destroy the works of the devil, and we can apply that directly to ourselves. Jesus manifests in our lives to destroy the works of the devil in us and in others! His love becomes our action. This is why Paul wrote, "And He Himself gave some to be apostles, some prophets, some evangelists, and some pastors and teachers, *for the equipping of the saints for the work of ministry*, for the edifying of the body of Christ" (Eph. 4:11–12, emphasis added).

Believers are meant to perform works of service. Jesus equips us to do them. It is the love walk. As T. L. Osborn writes,

> You are His co-worker. The emotions you feel are His emotions being reflected through you. It is God who is at work within you, giving you the will and the power to achieve his purpose (Philippians 2:13). One translation says: God is the energizer within you. The same one says: There are varieties of things accomplished but the same God does the energizing in them all (1 Corinthians 12:6). You say, "Now I will not only be fulfilled and happy myself; I will be able to do God's work." God is going to use all that He has created, which He declares is good, to bless you,

then to make you a blessing. Jesus said, The Father that dwells with me, he will do the work (John 14:10). God made the abundant good that surrounds you. He wills to use it to bless you and to bless others through you. You are hooked up with God to do the big kingdom business of blessing all who choose to believe. You have purpose. You have self-dignity. You experience a new birth of your own worth. You must have dominion because you are in union with God.[1]

Jim Bakker recently shared with us one of the most powerful moments he experienced while serving time in a federal prison. As some readers may remember, Jim and his wife, Tammy Faye Bakker, built one of the most multifaceted ministries in the world in the 1980s. Before that they helped pioneer the Trinity Broadcasting Network (TBN), worked with Pat Robertson at *The 700 Club*, and then launched their own television program, *The PTL Club*, which continued to break new ground in Christian media. The Bakkers envisioned and constructed Heritage USA, a 2,300-acre gathering place with highrise hotels and shops in South Carolina for Christians that at one time drew six million people per year for conferences and family-friendly entertainment.

All this came crashing down when a federal court wrongly found Jim guilty of mail fraud, wire fraud, and conspiring to defraud the public. He served five years of a forty-five-year sentence before Alan Dershowitz and other lawyers successfully appealed his case and Jim walked free.

One day during his time in prison, Jim was cleaning toilets when a prison guard came in.

"Bakker! You have a visitor," the guard announced.

"It's not visiting day," Jim said.

"You need to go to the warden's office right now," the guard said.

"I must be in trouble," Jim thought. "Nobody comes to visit me."

Jim had been cleaning toilets that day in spite of having pneumonia. He was wearing his grubby work clothes, including a pair of sneakers with holes in the toes. His hair was a mess, and he hadn't been allowed to comb it. He looked like a man who had been sleeping under a bridge. Disheveled, he made his way to the warden's office across the prison yard.

"Bakker, what are you doing here?" one guard barked.

"They called me to see the warden," Jim replied.

Then someone came out of the office and said, "Bakker, you have a visitor."

"It's not visiting day," Jim repeated. "Who is here?"

"Has nobody told you?" the office person said. "Billy Graham is here. Do you want to see him?"

Jim cast a glance down at himself. He was embarrassed by his appearance. Not only that, but the last time he had seen Billy Graham was when Billy was a guest on his television show back when *The PTL Club* was one of the most popular shows in Christian television.

"I don't want him to see me looking like this, but he came, so I have to," Jim thought.

He walked into the visiting room. Wardens and assistant wardens had gathered, all wanting to see Billy Graham. There stood the famous evangelist, towering over others at six feet three inches tall. By comparison, Jim was physically small. Billy saw him, stretched out his arms, walked over, and pulled Jim into a hug.

"Jim, I love you," he said.

Jim was so taken aback, he told us later. He had been disgraced in the eyes of the world, and yet here was one of the most respected men on the planet visiting him in prison, holding him in his arms, saying he loved him.

Jim began to protest. "No, I can't let you hug me. I've been cleaning toilets. I smell terrible."

"I am going to hug you, Jim. I love you," Billy said.

Billy was simply obeying what Jesus said: "I was in prison and you came to Me" (Matt. 25:36). Jim Bakker felt the love of God in his darkest hour because his friend Billy Graham went out of his way to put love into action.

ENVISIONING LOVING ACTIONS

I usually have to see something clearly before I can do it effectively.

Actions begin in the mind. We get a mental picture of what we want to do, and then we carry it out. When we read Scripture, it is no good if what we learn bears no fruit in our behavior. In other words, as we read the Word, we must see ourselves doing it. Our imagination turns into a planning center that produces a plan of action.

For example, I may find my attention especially drawn to a place in the Gospels where Jesus spoke words of life to someone or ministered to their need or ailment. So I picture myself doing the same thing in my own daily life. I keep that action in mind and go through my day looking for opportunities to carry it out. I might also picture myself driving peacefully in traffic and forgiving bad drivers before they cut me off! Maybe I picture myself doing something thoughtful for Mary, like bringing her flowers, or for my employees, or for someone else as I am led by the Holy Spirit. The Word says those who plan peace are blessed. This planning begins in the mind as we meditate on the Word and premeditate our acts of faith.

There are many biblical examples of visualizing acts of love and faithfulness. Jesus told His disciples, "Let us go into the next towns, that I may preach there also, because for this purpose I have come forth" (Mark 1:38). He had a vision for what He was going to do that day, and He carried it out. I believe David was visualizing success when he gathered five smooth stones from a creek bed. Paul wrote of his anticipation to visit the believers in Rome and then to be sent from there to other lands to preach where the gospel had not yet been heard (Rom. 15:23–24).

Doing always begins with envisioning. Once we have that love-driven vision, we put it into practice in real life. Paul said in Acts 24:16, "And herein do I exercise myself, to have always a conscience void to offence toward God, and toward men" (KJV). I love that word *exercise*. Working out our bodies is great, but we also have to exercise our love in all sorts of ways, putting patience, forgiveness, generosity, kindness, and faithfulness into practice.

Have you ever noticed that when Jesus healed people, He usually gave them something to do immediately? Jesus told some to get up, some to take their mats and go home. Others He commanded to show themselves to the priest, or to eat something, or to wash in a pool, or to preach to their hometown about the goodness of God. In this way, Jesus connected the healing power of His love to immediate obedience and action. He made the person exercise obedience to God's commands so the benefit of the miracle would not be lost over time. He was communicating that the benefits God provides are not one-and-done events. Rather, they happen and are sustained as we abide in the love of God and demonstrate our love for Him through obedience to His commands. This is why Jesus told one man He healed, "Sin no more, lest a worse thing come upon you" (John 5:14). Love must be exercised continually!

You may not want to love the "stinky" people in your path— the grumpy cashier, the rude driver, that relative you have a hard time getting along with. Just remember that back in Jesus' day there was no deodorant. He ministered all day long to people who seldom bathed and couldn't afford perfumes. The next time you read the Gospel accounts and come across a reference to a crowd, imagine the odor of sweat that must have emanated from them. If Jesus could abide the smelly, ungrateful people of His day, we should do no less. Spend time in His Word imagining ways to exercise your love, stay in the Spirit, follow the inner unction, and when He speaks, obey! We have within us the power of love that fashioned the universe, but it remains dormant until we do something with it (exercise or express it).

I try to face every decision I make by first running it through the love commandment. Before every word, I ask, Is it loving? The Holy Spirit is faithful to nudge me to indicate what action to perform or what words to say to express love in each circumstance. One thing I do consistently is hold the door for everyone. It doesn't matter who needs it or how many people I have to wait to pass through. If someone is coming, I hold the door. It has become a pleasure to me. On the other hand, I'm still learning to exercise love in the form of patience on highways when I get behind a slow driver, but I can do all things through Christ who strengthens me!

GRATITUDE

Earlier I wrote about how powerful it is to express gratitude. People who have great favor on their lives are usually the ones giving thanks all the time. They take nothing for granted.

The healthiest people also are thankful. An expert in the study of gratitude, Robert Emmons, wrote a book called *Thanks! How the New Science of Gratitude Can Make You Happier.* In it, he highlights key benefits of gratitude on our bodies and minds. They include the following:

- Psychological well-being: Practicing gratitude has been linked to improved psychological health, including reduced symptoms of depression and anxiety. "Grateful individuals tend to experience more positive emotions, greater life satisfaction, and increased resilience in the face of adversity," Emmons wrote.

- Physical health: Gratitude, said Emmons, has been linked to various physical health benefits, including better sleep quality, reduced inflammation, and improved cardiovascular health. His studies also show that people who regularly practice gratitude tend to engage in healthier behaviors and experience fewer physical symptoms of illness.

- Immune function: Emmons' research indicates that gratitude may have a positive impact on immune function. Grateful individuals have been found to exhibit stronger immune systems, which leads to better resistance against illness and faster recovery from illness or injury.

- Health behaviors: Interestingly, Emmons found that gratitude is associated with healthier lifestyle behaviors such as engaging in regular exercise, eating a balanced diet, and seeking preventive health care. Grateful individuals are more likely to prioritize self-care and engage in health-promoting activities.

- Overall well-being: Emmons' research suggests that cultivating gratitude is associated with higher levels of overall well-being and life satisfaction. Grateful individuals tend to experience greater levels of happiness, optimism, and a greater sense of meaning and purpose in life.[2]

Emmons defines gratitude this way: "Gratitude practice is systematically paying attention to what is going right in one's life, to see the contributions that others make in these good things, and then expressing gratitude verbally and behaviorally. Gratitude practice is intentionally shifting your attention from the negative to the positive and allowing your inner voice to speak that truth. Gratitude practice is acknowledging that even difficult and painful moments are our teachers and we can be grateful for them."[3]

Emmons notes that people who are thankful have a lower risk of developing chronic health conditions. They develop stronger relationships because gratitude fosters deeper connections and stronger bonds with others. And expressing appreciation, he wrote, can increase feelings of trust and intimacy and promote social support networks.[4]

IT'S A FACT!

In one study, people who practiced gratitude reported feeling closer to others. They also experienced lower levels of stress and negative emotions, indicating that thankfulness protects against daily stress and its corrosive health effects. Practicing gratitude was associated with better physical health outcomes, such as fewer symptoms of illness and greater overall health. When participants kept daily gratitude journals, recording things they were grateful for in addition to troublesome experiences, they elevated their well-being and overall quality of life.[5]

Many Christians read scriptures about thankfulness and think they only mean to express thankfulness toward God. But when the Bible commands us to express thanks, it also means expressing it to one another. This adds to the impact of verses such as "in everything give thanks; for this is the will of God in Christ Jesus for you" (1 Thess. 5:18). In everything we must give thanks to God and to people.

After all we've learned about gratitude and kindness thus far, perhaps it will come as no surprise that "positive communication within romantic relationships [has an] impact on sexual and relationship satisfaction." A study conducted by California State University, Chico, using data from 246 couples, "explore[d] how expressions of affection, compliments, and fondness contribute to the satisfaction and desire among partners....The study revealed that positive communication, encompassing acts like showing affection and giving compliments, consistently leads to higher levels of satisfaction and desire in relationships for both individuals and their partners."[6]

Mary and I have taken this principle to heart, and we look for reasons to thank each other for little things.

"Don, thanks for taking the trash out. That means I don't have to," Mary will tell me.

"Thanks for making this breakfast," I tell her.

We also give thanks to servers at restaurants, clerks at airport counters and grocery stores, and anyone else we come in contact with. We acknowledge them by name and tip them for their good service. Appreciation is a major part of the love walk. It works against our own sense of entitlement; it focuses us on the value of the people around us and the services they perform. When we give thanks in all things, God adds things to be thankful for.

BECOMING GIVERS

Love also serves others, as Galatians 5:13 (NLT) says: "Use your freedom to serve one another in love." Jesus is quoted in Acts 20:35 as having said, "It is more blessed to give than to receive" (NLT). How does Jesus love you? By giving! In John 15:13 Jesus said, "Greater love has no one than this, than to lay down one's life for his friends." In John 3:16 He said, "For God so loved the world that He *gave* His only begotten Son, that whoever believes in Him should not perish but have everlasting life" (emphasis added).

First John 3:16–18 says, "By this we know love, because He laid down His life for us. And we also ought to lay down our lives for the brethren. But whoever has this world's goods and sees his brother in need, and shuts up his heart from him, how does the love of God abide in him? My little children, let us not love in word or in tongue, but in deed and in truth."

God shows love by giving, and the Bible tells us as His

children to excel in the grace of giving as well (2 Cor. 8:7). We are happier and therefore healthier when we are blessed, and we are more blessed when we give. This is God's equation, and it works every time.

The church in its early days abounded in joy by giving freely to those among them in need. Acts 2:44–45 says, "Now all who believed were together, and had all things in common, and sold their possessions and goods, and divided them among all, as anyone had need."

If the church today lived in a spirit of generosity like that, there would be an explosion of evangelism and growth. The gospel would spread like a wildfire in a prairie wind. Those early Christians were carrying out Jesus' command, "By this all will know that you are My disciples, if you have love for one another" (John 13:35). To love is to give whenever and whatever the Lord leads us to give.

What are some practical ways to give? Jesus gave us direction in Matthew 25:35–36:

> For I was hungry and you gave Me food; I was thirsty and you gave Me drink; I was a stranger and you took Me in; I was naked and you clothed Me; I was sick and you visited Me; I was in prison and you came to Me.

When was the last time you gave someone food or something to drink or welcomed a new person into your community or home? When have you given someone clothes or shoes or visited someone in the hospital or in prison? These are basic measures of generosity, and of course there are many other ways to give as well. Gary Chapman wrote a best-selling book called *The 5 Love Languages* that helpfully identifies five common expressions of love. They are:

1. Quality time

2. Giving gifts

3. Words of affirmation

4. Acts of service

5. Physical touch

Love discovers which expressions the people around us appreciate, then envisions and carries out appropriate acts of love.

Whatever you do, put love into action. I often think of Bill Bright, one of the great men I have known, who was my patient for years. For about a year I went to his house almost every Wednesday night for a house call. Mary and I called it "Bright night" because every time I went, I got more out of it than Bill did! He was one of the greatest examples of love I have ever personally known. Most people from his generation know that his ministry, Campus Crusade for Christ, now called CRU, brought an estimated 150 million people to Christ—and counting. Bill was so passionate about reaching the lost and loving God that he pioneered doing forty-day fasts, sometimes fasting on water alone. Whenever I went into his house, the presence of God felt overwhelming.

As he was dying with pulmonary fibrosis, Bill still worked like he was a young man. He pulled two beds together and spread out ten or so manuscripts on which he was working at the same time. Fighting for breath, his lungs scarred, he told me excitedly, "Look at this manuscript. This book is going to be called *Till My Last Breath*."

I really do believe I saw Jesus in his eyes. I have rarely seen love pour out of someone's eyes like that. The only other time

I've witnessed it was when a friend of mine went to heaven and came back to tell about it.

One day I was there at the house when Bill's wife, Vonette, told him, "Bill, I'm so sorry you have to suffer." Bill looked at her like she had lost her mind.

"Suffer?" he said. "I'm not suffering. Jesus suffered. He wore the crown of thorns, was lashed thirty-nine times, was nailed to a cross. He suffered."

That was Bill's mindset, and he worked in the strength of God's love to the end of his days to get the Word out. Like Bill, each of us will stand before God on the day of judgment and give an account of our acts of love on this earth—so let's make every opportunity count.

In the next chapter we will look at what I believe is the single most important action we can take to walk in God's love.

PRAYER AND DECLARATIONS

Father God, I commit to love with words and with deeds. I will be a doer and exerciser of love! You live in me, and You are perfect love; therefore, I will behave in a loving way in all things. I will act and react with patience and kindness, letting Your love flow from my heart toward others. Lord, help me to grasp and put into practice the many ways love expresses itself. Thank You for the privilege of growing in love so I look more like You! Amen.

I will not allow myself to be envious or boil over with jealousy. I will not be boastful or vainglorious nor display myself haughtily. Rather, I will act in godly humility, considering others better than myself.

Love is not rude or unmannerly and does not act in an unbecoming way, so neither do I.

I will practice generosity and kindness everywhere I go today—in my home, in public places, on the streets and highways.

I will not insist on my own rights or my own way, for love is not self-seeking. I am not selfish; instead, I put others' desires before my own.

I will not be touchy, fretful, or resentful, and I will take no account of the evil done to me.

I will not rejoice at injustice or unrighteousness, sin, ungodliness, rebellion, or wickedness but rejoice when right and truth prevail.

I will endeavor to bear up under anything and everything that comes my way, always ready to believe the best of every person. I will exercise love that endures without weakening.

The Comforter, the Holy Spirit, lives in me and enables me to endure everything.

Love never fails, fades, or becomes obsolete. It is always effective, so I never need to quit.

SECTION II:
FREEDOM FROM TORMENTORS

CHAPTER 6

FORGIVING: THE KEY TO LIVING

MARY AND I were in Canada many years ago doing publicity for one of my books, and while there we visited the home of the couple whose ministry was hosting us. This family outwardly seemed to be doing well. The couple's daughter and son-in-law had four young children, including a newborn, and between their growing brood and successful ministry the parents should have been rejoicing in all the Lord was doing. But that night as we fellowshipped with them and others, Mary and I noticed a great heaviness in their home. The son-in-law's health issues kept coming up in conversation, so I finally offered to check him out. It didn't take long for me to conclude that he was full of bitterness, which was ravaging his health. "What on earth is going on here?" I wondered.

Totally ignorant of their situation, I announced perhaps a little abruptly, "You are full of bitterness. Who are you angry at, and what happened?"

It was one of those moments when the whole room goes quiet. I felt like I had stepped on a land mine that was about to explode. Then the man's wife spoke up.

"I had an affair on my husband and got pregnant," she said. "This new baby is from that affair."

Whoa! The impact of her words was palpable—and not easy to hear. It certainly explained why the baby had such noticeably different skin and hair color from the other children. The biological father of this child, she said, was an eighteen-year-old man from another country who had been staying with them in their house and working for their Christian business. When the wife found out she was pregnant, she told the young man, "You have to leave now and go back to where you're from, because I have to tell my husband about this tonight, and I don't know what will happen." The young man complied, which probably forestalled a very bad situation.

When she confessed the affair to her husband, the next words out of her mouth stunned her, as a Christian: "Do you want me to have an abortion? If that is what you want me to do, I am willing," she told him.

The husband, though suffering all the horrible emotions imaginable with this situation, replied, "One wrong does not correct another wrong. We are not doing that. We will work with this situation, but we are not killing the baby."

To make it more complex, the husband had undergone a vasectomy, which everybody in their community of friends and colleagues knew about, and so the wife's pregnancy was clearly going to raise suspicions. To protect his family from speculations and shame, the husband moved them all to Phoenix for the pregnancy and birth.

Their marriage was in tatters as the couple tried to move forward without trust or unity. Tommy Barnett's church, now called Dream City Church, took them in, ministered to them, and played a big part in trying to save their marriage. But for a while the man was considering the biblical option of leaving his wife and starting over with someone else. His heart was overcome with pain and feelings of betrayal. During that time in Arizona, however, he had an experience with Jesus that convinced him to stay with the family.

One evening he brought his wife and kids together in the living room. "I need to tell you something," he said to the children. "Mommy has done something, and she is very sorry for what she has done. Mommy is going to have a baby, but it is not from Daddy. It is from someone else. But I also want you to know that Daddy has decided to go through this situation like Jesus does with us."

He then took a blanket and put it over his pregnant wife.

"As Jesus covers our sins, Daddy has decided to cover her sin," he said.

It was an amazing display of mercy, and he stuck to his decision to keep the family together and forgive his wife. The baby was born, and he named him after himself, giving the child his own first name and making him a "junior." He explained, "Jesus adopted us and gave us His name. He asked me to do the same thing He did for me."

MIRACLE BREAKTHROUGH

The family returned to Canada, but walking through the aftereffects of deep pain and betrayal proved difficult over time. The couple had never regained their intimacy. Bitterness raged within the man's soul as he grappled with the situation his wife had put them in and the emotional suffering she had caused him. That was around the time Mary and I visited Canada and stumbled into this scenario. We were flabbergasted by numerous elements of their story, and as a medical professional and brother in the Lord I didn't know what else to do but offer to walk them through steps of forgiveness, which I knew might help.

"I'm not ready for that," the husband said quickly, adding that he still felt he wanted to divorce her. But the wife said, "I would like to try." In another room, in the presence of Mary and the husband, I started leading her through the steps. She had such a hard time forgiving herself for what she had done but finally experienced a real breakthrough and grabbed hold of God's mercy for her. After a while I turned to the husband to see if he had changed his mind.

"I can do this for you too, and you can be free," I offered very gently. "We'll be here a few days more. I can assure you that for you to get better spiritually and physically, at some point you will have to let go of this bitterness."

"Let me pray about it," he said noncommittally.

The next night, Mary and I were getting ready to head back home to Florida. We and others were gathered in this couple's living room to say farewell, when the husband unexpectedly spoke up.

"I want to go through the steps of forgiveness," he said. "I want to be free."

And so I began taking him through the steps of forgiveness. He broke and started sobbing, then turned to his wife, grabbed her, and said, "I forgive you!" She clung to him, and they collapsed to the floor, both weeping rivers of tears. We watched this incredibly powerful moment—a true relational miracle—take place in that living room.

I'm happy to say that twenty years later, this couple has ministered to thousands of people, written books together, and held marriage seminars all over the country. The wonderful work of restoration God did in their marriage and family has encouraged so many others to press through terrible circumstances. The forgiveness the husband was able to offer gave hope to every couple torn apart by betrayal. It was a demonstration of the power of God's mercy. If this couple, raising a child born of an affair as their own beloved son, could make it, anyone could. Their book *Marriage Under Cover* tells their full story.

Quit Picking

Of all the actions we take in the love walk, forgiveness is by far the most important. Lack of forgiveness is the main hindrance to people experiencing the full health benefits of abiding in the Lord.

In my office, we often have patients come in who are "scab pickers." They can't control themselves from relentlessly picking any scab that forms on their bodies. For example, one man got a little scratch from a thorny bush while he was doing yard work. It wasn't anything bad, but he kept picking the scab off, causing it to bleed, and eventually it became infected. This led to a staph infection that required IV antibiotics to clear up. Those powerful antibiotics caused a lot of problems for his body—and it all began with his incessant picking of a relatively small scab.

Bitterness is like that—pulling a scab off and reopening a wound so it never heals. It is often said that bitterness is like drinking poison and expecting the other person (who offended or violated us) to die. Our bodies are not meant to harbor bitterness. It consumes the container it is in, like putting hydrochloric acid in a plastic cup. We are not made to hold it. Yet so many people are stuck in offense, singing every refrain of the "Somebody Done Me Wrong" song. I have watched Christians carry bitterness wounds for thirty years or more. You can see it etched on their faces and foreheads, hear it in their attitudes and speech, and witness the effects in their relationships. Bitterness is ruinous of their mental and physical health, because while our bodies and minds are meant to function for brief periods of time in emergency mode—if we are running from a Rottweiler, for example, or escaping a fire—the emergency chemicals released by bitterness and its accompanying emotions will eventually invite disease in or kill us over time.

Unforgiveness causes the body to go into a hypervigilant state in which it secretes too much cortisol (similar to cortisone) and adrenaline, causing blood vessels to stay constricted. This sets up the alarm and resistance stage of the stress response. The body is hardwired to react to stress this way, but the responses that save our lives when we are attacked begin to harm and eventually destroy our bodies when sustained for more than short bursts. They may cause tension headaches, anxiety, chronic muscle tension, and immune system dysregulation, leading to excessive inflammation, autoimmune disease, or a weakened immune response. Nobody was designed to be fleeing or fighting all the time.

Dr. Fred Luskin, a prominent psychologist, has extensively researched the impact of forgiveness on happiness, health, and overall well-being. His work, particularly through the Stanford Forgiveness Project, has shed light on the profound effects of forgiveness on various aspects of our lives. Luskin emphasizes that holding on to grudges and resentment can lead to stress, anxiety, and negative emotions, while offering forgiveness can have numerous benefits.

"Fascinating research has emerged in the past ten years that documents the healing power of forgiveness," Luskin wrote.

"Forgiveness training has been shown to reduce depression, increase hopefulness, decrease anger, improve spiritual connection, increase emotional self-confidence, and help heal relationships. Learning to forgive is good for both your mental and physical well-being and your relationships."[1] According to Luskin's research:

- People who forgive have fewer health issues.
- Forgiveness reduces stress and its physical symptoms.
- Holding grudges may pose a greater heart disease risk than hostility.
- Blaming others increases the likelihood of heart disease, cancer, and other illnesses.
- Unforgiving thoughts can negatively affect blood pressure, muscle tension, and immunity.
- Forgiving thoughts can quickly improve cardiovascular, muscular, and nervous system health.[2]

Forgiveness, Luskin wrote, can lead to reduced levels of anger, which is significant because holding on to anger and resentment has been linked to various health problems, including hypertension, heart disease, and weakened immune function. By contrast, forgiveness can lower stress levels and promote better cardiovascular health.[3]

A study conducted by Luskin and others used a randomized trial to study the effects of "group forgiveness intervention," which aimed to help participants forgive others and reduce their levels of stress and anger. They found that participants who forgave better experienced reduced perceived stress and decreased anger compared to those who held on to resentment.[4]

Forgiveness is also associated with enhanced immune functioning. Participants in another study who reported higher levels of forgiveness also had higher CD4 counts, an indicator of a stronger immune system, compared to those who reported lower levels of forgiveness.[5]

Yet many people choose to live with unresolved bitterness. A Fetzer Institute study in 2010 found that 62 percent of Americans confessed to needing more forgiveness in their personal lives. A 2022 survey of two thousand adults by Trustpilot's Helping Hands found that 69 percent held a grudge toward someone, with the worst offenders being those who live in the Midwest.[6]

But the truth is that everyone is tempted to open the door at times to the torment that bitterness brings.

An Open Door to Tormentors

While the effects of unforgiveness always manifest in our physical bodies, they actually originate in the realm of the spirit. This is because while forgiveness allows God to freely move and abide in our lives, lack of forgiveness opens the door to the activity of literal tormentors. Jesus described these tormentors and how they get access to our lives:

> Then Peter came to Him and said, "Lord, how often shall my brother sin against me, and I forgive him? Up to seven times?" Jesus said to him, "I do not say to you, up to seven times, but up to seventy times seven."
>
> —Matthew 18:21–22

For context, in Old Testament times people were only required to forgive a repeat offense three times based on Amos 1 and 2. But Jesus said to forgive seventy times seven times, and not just over the course of a lifetime but in one day. In other words, we are to cultivate a constant willingness to forgive. Jesus then illustrated this kingdom truth by telling what is often referred to as the parable of the unmerciful servant.

> Therefore the kingdom of heaven is like a certain king who wanted to settle accounts with his servants. And when he had begun to settle accounts, one was brought to him who owed him ten thousand talents.
>
> —MATTHEW 18:23–24

Ten thousand talents would be billions of dollars in today's money. To pay off one talent, you would have had to work six thousand days. To pay off ten thousand talents, you would have had to work sixty million days, an impossible debt. Jesus continued:

> But as he was not able to pay, his master commanded that he be sold, with his wife and children and all that he had, and that payment be made. The servant therefore fell down before him, saying, "Master, have patience with me, and I will pay you all." Then the master of that servant was moved with compassion, released him, and forgave him the debt.
>
> —MATTHEW 18:25–27

> But that servant went out and found one of his fellow servants who owed him a hundred denarii; and he laid hands on him and took him by the throat, saying, "Pay me what you owe!"
>
> —MATTHEW 18:28

Pence is another word for a denarius, and one hundred pence equals one hundred days of work.

So his fellow servant fell down at his feet and begged him, saying, "Have patience with me, and I will pay you all." And he would not, but went and threw him into prison till he should pay the debt. So when his fellow servants saw what had been done, they were very grieved, and came and told their master all that had been done. Then his master, after he had called him, said to him, "You wicked servant! I forgave you all that debt because you begged me. Should you not also have had compassion on your fellow servant, just as I had pity on you?" And his master was angry, and delivered him to the torturers until he should pay all that was due to him.

So My heavenly Father also will do to you if each of you, from his heart, does not forgive his brother his trespasses.

—MATTHEW 18:29–35

The final words of that story, spoken by Jesus' own mouth, are incredibly chilling: "So My heavenly Father also will do to you." The King James Version calls the entities mentioned in verse 34 "tormentors," while the NKJV uses the similar term "torturers." I asked my friend Rick Renner, a great Greek scholar, who the tormentors are in this parable. He said what I already believed: They are demons who put tormenting conditions and diseases on people. These illnesses include depression, cancer, fibromyalgia, chronic pain conditions, autoimmune conditions, rheumatoid arthritis, and much more.

When we are unmerciful and withhold our forgiveness, we give evil spirits legal authority to torment our bodies and minds. This is graphically depicted in the parable. It also sheds a whole new light on the fact that about half the miracles Jesus performed during His earthly ministry were to cast out spirits of infirmity, which resulted in physical healing. Evil spirits had gained legal access to the minds and bodies of people and proceeded to torment them, sometimes for decades! Jesus did not just heal people's bodies; He cast out the tormentors who were causing the diseases and dysfunctions.

IT'S A FACT!

Forgiveness is not a feeling; it's a choice to obey the Lord and cancel the perceived debt someone owes you. Love keeps no record of being wronged, according to 1 Corinthians 13:5 (NLT), so we should throw away the record-keeping book.

This is a well-established biblical reality. John the apostle wrote that "fear involves torment" (1 John 4:18), meaning that fear is not just a negative emotion but a literal open door for the tormentors. When we agree with fear, we welcome spirits into our minds and emotions to torment us. Paul wrote about this in Galatians 5:15, one of the most powerful scriptures in the whole Bible on this topic. Bitterness and strife open the door for demons to work.

> But if you bite and devour one another, beware lest you be consumed by one another!
>
> —GALATIANS 5:15

> For where envying and strife is, there is confusion and every evil work.
>
> —JAMES 3:16, KJV

What a vivid and alarming word picture about how strife consumes people—eating up their time, energy, and relationships, and causing them to consume one another. When we open the door to him, the enemy feasts on us and uses us to feast on others.

Paul told another church that he had turned some rebellious people over to Satan for the salvation of their souls because they had opened the door to the enemy's ongoing influence (1 Tim. 1:20). These men chose to allow tormentors into their minds, so Paul allowed them to suffer the consequences with the hope that they would repent and return to the Lord and to fellowship with other Christians.

When Christians abide in bitterness rather than walk the love walk, we quench the Holy Spirit—another way of saying we close the door to His influence and open it instead to the tormentors. This is why the Bible exhorts us to put off the old man with its fleshly desires (Eph. 4:22), to have this mind in us which was also in Christ Jesus (Phil. 2:5), and many other such commands. Paul is describing a lifestyle in which we give God ongoing access and influence in our lives by an act of our will and at the same time shut the door to tormenting spirits by staying in the love walk, chiefly by forgiving others.

Think for a moment if there are areas where you feel tormented. Whose influence are you allowing in your mind and body? Who is living through you in your thoughts or behaviors? Is it possible you have opened the door to tormentors and their destructive toolkit of illnesses and dysfunctions? It is time to evict those tormentors by forgiving and getting back into the love walk!

SIGNING UP FOR FIBROMYALGIA

A woman came into my office one day with severe, stage III kidney disease. She had suffered with diabetes and hypertension for years, and I knew that if I didn't get her blood pressure down, she was heading toward dialysis. As I took her health history, I recognized symptoms of past abandonment. So I asked her with some confidence, "Do you have abandonment issues? Did something happen in your younger years to make you feel abandoned?"

Her husband, who was with her in my office, piped up: "She had an abortion."

The woman nodded to acknowledge it was true.

"Do you want to go through forgiveness therapy, to forgive yourself according to Ephesians 4:32 and break off deadly emotions flowing from that?" I asked her.

Essentially, I was asking if she wanted to kick out the tormentors who had access to her mind and body.

"Yes," she agreed, and within minutes I led her through prayers and statements that helped to break negative strongholds that had bound her for years. This woman's appearance and entire demeanor transformed before our very eyes, and the husband was nothing short of amazed. He got his wife back that day.

IT'S A FACT!

Researchers have found that "grudges created negative emotions and intrusive thoughts that impacted quality of life. Given the negative experience of holding onto a grudge, why do people do so? Based on the qualitative findings across three studies…three factors emerged: disdain (dislike, intolerance) for the transgressor; emotional persistence (sustained feelings of anger, hurt); and perceived longevity (the sense of never being able to let go of the grudge)."[7]

This woman's health greatly improved as a result of shutting out the tormentors, but what sometimes haunts me about her situation and many others is that for so many years in my medical practice I did not recognize the role of remaining in the love walk to sustain health and vitality. I gave many patients a powerful slice of the truth—teaching them to forgive people by an act of the will, helping them to avoid toxic emotions and stress, attacking their problems from a clinical point of view— but I did not lead them deep into the river of God's love, which makes it so much easier to live completely free of tormenting problems. I had not yet connected ultimate health and wellness to abiding in the love that flows freely from the throne of God.

I mentioned earlier that a shocking 69 percent of Americans surveyed in 2022 indicated they felt lingering resentment from a range of experiences, such as job rejections, relationship setbacks, and poor consumer interactions, according to a report on the survey in *Forbes*. "Although 70% acknowledged that it was harmful to their health to hold onto a grudge, about the same percentage admitted to harboring a grudge."[8] The same poll found that most people hold on to a grudge for five years at the longest, but 15 percent had held on to a grudge for eleven or more years.[9]

The authors concluded that no matter how strong the urge is to hold on to grudges, the best thing to do is find a way to let them go. "Forgiveness may be the best antidote to the psychological toxins created by grudges, such as negative rumination, bitterness, resentment, anger, depression, and anxiety," they wrote.[10] A large body of psychological research suggests that the difficult work of doing so yields positive benefits.

PUT AWAY SELF-HATRED AND REGRET

Over twenty years ago a woman who was the worst fibromyalgia patient I've ever seen came into my office. She was obese and had many other health issues, including high blood pressure, insomnia, depression, diabetes, and anxiety. Her muscles were as hard as rocks.

"When did all this start?" I asked.

"About ten years ago," she answered.

"What happened ten years ago?"

"My husband started having an affair with my best friend," she began. "That woman's husband found out about it, came over, and beat my husband so severely that he had to go into intensive care at the hospital. I would come visit my husband every day, but my best friend was also coming by to visit him, and I heard the nurses whispering and laughing about this. One day I went there and he was gone. He had left with my best friend."

It was as if a dump truck had pulled up and unloaded every bad emotion on this woman: abandonment, betrayal, rejection, grief, humiliation, hatred of herself and everyone around her. Like many misused and abused women I've treated, she had built a wall of protection around herself by gaining weight on purpose so men would not prey on her anymore. The extra pounds were her perceived protection—but the resentment fueling her problems would eventually kill her.

She was trapped in a prison of self-hatred. She hated herself for being gullible and falling victim to this betrayal and rejection by the two closest people in her life. Almost every auto-immune disease has a root cause of self-hatred. If people do not love themselves as Jesus commanded them to, their bodies may eventually turn on themselves. The body is obedient to our spirits. If we hold a hostile view of ourselves, the body may eventually treat itself with hostility. If we store up anger and bitterness toward others, the mind has nowhere to store it but within ourselves, and so we become the receptacle of our own poisons.

I took this woman through the process of forgiveness, and she was set free. Her muscles relaxed, and everything got better. She broke the cycle of death she had been stuck in due to unrelenting self-hatred and bitterness toward others.

This kind of situation happens all the time in my practice, especially with fibromyalgia patients who suffer from severe pain and are taking multiple medications but usually still have not gotten better. They almost always have unforgiveness buried somewhere inside, often directed toward both themselves and others. Once they step out of that cycle and embark on the love walk, their stress response usually is turned off, they start sleeping again, and their pain usually diminishes and disappears. It's amazing.

Toss Out the Rearview Mirror

Regret is an exceedingly harmful emotion. In Luke 9:62 Jesus warned us not to fixate on the past, saying, "No one, having put his hand to the plow, and looking back, is fit for the kingdom of God." That gives us a picture of regret—walking in one direction, stepping into a new work, new ministries, new frontiers, new relationships, then looking back and losing effectiveness, drifting off God's chosen path for our future.

Have you ever looked over your shoulder too long while driving a car or riding a bike? The tendency is to veer in that direction because of what is called visual-directional control. That is the technique used to train fighter pilots: Put your eyes where you want to go and the rest of you will follow. When we look back, we end up going in circles, getting nowhere.

Paul wrote words we can apply directly to our lives:

> Brethren, I do not count myself to have apprehended; but one thing I do, forgetting those things which are behind and reaching forward to those things which are ahead, I press toward the goal for the prize of the upward call of God in Christ Jesus.
>
> —PHILIPPIANS 3:13–14

Notice that the goal, the prize, the upward call of God is always in front of us. What do we do about the stuff behind us? God commands us to forget it! It can only take us backward and cause us to be mired in regret. Paul easily could have allowed himself to get stuck in the past due to his many mistakes and unjust sufferings. But his strategy—and it worked out pretty well for his ministry—was to "press toward" what God had for him in the future. He ripped off the rear-view mirror and threw it away.

I was impressed by what I read about Mother Teresa, the renowned servant of the poorest street people in Calcutta, India. "Mother Teresa saw bitterness as a major obstacle to love and an impediment to one's spiritual life," this book read. "Unwillingness to forgive results in resentment and bitterness or a desire for revenge....Sensitive by nature, Mother Teresa suffered keenly from hurts, but she was determined not to let them control or influence her choices. Instead of focusing on herself, she focused on the person who hurt her, actually feeling sorry for them because she knew that in reality they were hurting themselves more than her. By her forgiveness, she offered everyone the opportunity to start anew."[11]

As God practices forgetfulness, so we must practice forget-fulness with ourselves and others. Isaiah 43:25 tells us that God does not remember our sins, so what gives us the right to keep dragging them out for inspection? It is the best news possible that we are not supposed to remember our own sins! We are set free from keeping account of what we have done wrong.

Hebrews 10:17 says, with God speaking, "Their sins and their lawless deeds I will remember no more." Who are we to bring them up again? The constant cataloging only keeps us stuck in self-hatred. It sets a table of poison in front of us, and we eat of it. God does not feed us the food of self-hatred. Rather, He presents a feast for us in the presence of our enemies! Many are eating the wrong banquet, by choice.

I speak strongly about this because self-hatred is such a sin-ister, self-justifying attitude that people allow to exist within themselves. They think they need to keep reminding them-selves of their terrible past, the mistakes they made, the harm they did to their own lives or the lives of others. The enemy keeps bringing it up to them, and they get depressed all over again. They can't escape from themselves. It is literally a demonic trap—and in the next chapter I will expose one of the more deceptive ways the enemy maneuvers us into this trap and out of the love walk. But first let's pray and declare!

PRAYER AND DECLARATIONS

Father, I no longer want to sign up for diseases and mental torment due to bitterness and holding grudges! It is not justified, and I ask You to forgive me for allowing that root to corrupt my soul. By a deliberate act of my will, I release anyone who has harmed me from whatever I thought they owed me. I allow them to walk free so I can walk free! Help me as I continue to choose to forgive day by day, walking deeper in the love walk and becoming more like You, the author of mercy. Amen.

I will not pick at sensitive areas and wounds in my soul but will let God heal them with the balm of His love. I repent of revisiting and reopening old wounds.

I have the ability to forgive by an act of my will—and I know God will empower my decision with a flood of His grace, enabling me to release all bitterness and walk in newness of life, day by day.

I choose to forgive and forget those hurts and offenses from the past and evict the tormentors as I walk in love.

CHAPTER 7

CLEANSING OUR CONSCIENCES

L ET ME EXPOSE one of the enemy's most devious and effective strategies to drain the power from our lives. After causing us to look back in regret and leave the love walk, he then partners with our own consciences to condemn us for leaving it! In this way he uses our God-given internal compasses against us. Our consciences are designed to keep us in the love walk, but the enemy twists the signals they are sending and interprets them as condemning us.

God graciously endowed every human being with an internal guidance system called the conscience. It's an internal security system that sounds the alarm whenever we step out of the love walk and harbor deadly emotions such as bitterness, lust, envy, anger, and any other sinful attitude or behavior. Our consciences blare at us to quit the offending behavior and jump back into the river of God's love. As John the apostle put it, "our heart condemns us" (1 John 3:20). If we don't repent of the wrong we are doing, we begin to feel shame, blame, and guilt instead of love, peace, joy, and so on. Our hearts condemn us because our consciences are trying to rescue us from the tormentors. Love and condemnation do not work together. One has to go; the other will reign supreme.

This is why Paul wrote so often about the conscience. One time he was giving his testimony, and "looking earnestly at the council, [he] said, 'Men and brethren, I have lived in all good *conscience* before God until this day'" (Acts 23:1, emphasis added). On another occasion he said, "I myself always strive to have a *conscience* without offense toward God and men" (Acts 24:16, emphasis added). In his letter to the Romans, he said even people who have not yet heard the gospel have experienced a level of God-given awareness of the principles of righteousness, "their *conscience* also bearing witness, and between themselves their thoughts accusing or else excusing them" (Rom. 2:15, emphasis added).

He wrote about being subject to ruling authorities "for conscience' sake" and about brothers and sisters in the Lord who have a "weak conscience" (Rom. 13:5; 1 Cor. 8:12). He wrote of having a "good conscience," a "pure conscience" (1 Tim. 1:5; 3:9), and even said, "But we have renounced the hidden things of shame, not walking in craftiness nor handling the word of God deceitfully, but by manifestation of the truth commending ourselves to every man's *conscience* in the sight of God" (2 Cor. 4:2, emphasis added). It is possible to "sear" our consciences and to "cleanse" them (1 Tim. 4:2; Heb. 9:14). It is possible to have an "evil" conscience—that is, one made accustomed to wrongdoing (Heb. 10:22). Peter wrote of the nobility of believers suffering unjustly, "For this is commendable, if because of *conscience* toward God one endures grief, suffering wrongfully" (1 Pet. 2:19, emphasis added).

The work of our consciences is good, but when the enemy is able to warp what our consciences are telling us, turning them from a righteous warning to a merciless judgment, he employs God's own weapon against our minds and bodies. This quickly turns to self-hatred, which erodes the health of even committed Christians.

One study published in *Psychological Reports* looked at the effect of self-directed compassion on the relationship between bitterness and depression. More than three hundred participants completed a questionnaire that assessed their forgiveness, the level of grace and love they held toward themselves, and their levels of depressive symptoms. Results showed that the more compassion and forgiveness we hold toward ourselves, the less depression we experience and the easier we find it to forgive others.

IT'S A FACT!

Learning to love (and forgive) yourself is not just a biblical concept; it also has psychological benefits that have been the subject of rigorous study: "Self-compassion may help an individual feel positive emotions and view their painful feelings with understanding, kindness, and a sense of shared humanity which may allow them to forgive more easily."[1]

The authors of that study had discovered a biblical truth: that the antidote for self-condemnation is confidence toward God. A powerful passage in 1 John 3:20–24 (KJV) shines a bold light on the method of escape from this deceptive plan.

> For if our heart condemn us, God is greater than our heart, and knoweth all things. Beloved, if our heart condemn us not, then have we confidence toward God. And whatsoever we ask, we receive of him, because we keep his commandments, and do those things that are pleasing in

his sight. And this is his commandment, that we should believe on the name of his Son Jesus Christ, and love one another, as he gave us commandment. And he that keepeth his commandments dwelleth in him, and he in him. And hereby we know that he abideth in us, by the Spirit which he hath given us.

Notice the specific steps to overcoming this common problem:

1. We recognize that our hearts are condemning us.

2. We declare that God is greater than our hearts and knows everything.

3. We have confidence toward God.

4. We know that we will receive any good thing we ask of Him.

5. Our part of the deal is to walk the love walk by keeping His commandments and doing the things that are pleasing in His sight.

6. The primary ways of staying in the love walk are believing in Jesus Christ and loving each other.

7. By keeping these commands, we dwell in Him, and He in us.

8. We know for certain that He abides in us because we have His Spirit.

As a result, we stop experiencing needless condemnation from our consciences!

This is an amazing way to banish the enemy's accusations and a powerful principle we can apply in many areas of our lives daily. If you have fallen into a cycle of condemnation, holding on to bitterness and self-hatred (or any other sinful habit), then instead of entertaining fiery darts of the devil—which encourage resentful thoughts—cast those thoughts out. Philippians 4:6–8 says we are not allowed to worry about anything. If a thought occurs to us that does not conform to the qualifications of the love walk, cast it out! Do not tolerate it for one minute.

MEDICAL BENEFITS OF RELEASING BITTERNESS

Multiple studies have confirmed the life-giving effects of forgiving ourselves and others and the fact that bitterness is disastrous for the body, mind, and emotions. In a paper titled "Inflammation: The Common Pathway of Stress-Related Diseases," the authors wrote that, according to medical research, as much as 75 to 90 percent of illness and disease is stress-related.[2] That is a remarkable statement!

Bitterness causes stress, and stress interferes with normal, healthy body processes. Stress hormones can inhibit a process called anoikis, which kills diseased cells and prevents them from spreading. That means when we harbor grudges, disease gains a greater foothold in our bodies. Chronic stress also increases the production of certain growth factors that increase in our blood supply, which can speed the development of cancerous tumors.[3]

We literally decide moment by moment what our physical health will be. Approximately fifteen minutes after the onset of stress, cortisol levels rise, and they remain elevated for several hours.[4]

Stress can also enhance weight gain and fat deposition through changes in feeding behavior. Chronic stress is known to alter the patterns of how people eat, their dietary preference, and the rewarding properties of foods.[5]

When we entertain stressful thoughts, we shape our mental and physical health. It's as simple as that. But when we flood our minds with thoughts of mercy and forgiveness, it enhances our health in every regard. Luskin described the first study to specifically examine how forgiveness improves physical health. It showed that "when people think about forgiving an offender it leads to improved functioning in their cardiovascular and nervous systems." College students were asked to imagine that they had forgiven someone who had wronged them. They were told to actively give up thoughts of revenge against that person and choose an attitude of goodwill. The architects of the study prescribed periods of imagining forgiveness along with the periods of rehearsing grudges. When rehearsing grudges, "the subjects' blood pressure, heart rate, and arterial wall pressure all rose," Luskin writes. "These are negative experiences for one's cardiovascular system. If these responses occur for too long they can damage the heart and blood vessels."

> In addition, during the period of unforgiving imagery participants' muscle tension increased and the students reported feeling uncomfortable and less in control. During the forgiveness condition, there were no physiological disturbances and the students reported greater feelings of positive emotion and relaxation. This study exposed that both forgiveness and holding a grudge generate immediate physical and emotional reactions. The reactions were experienced as positive in the forgiveness condition and negative in the grudge condition. This study showed that holding a grudge in the short run could stress participants' nervous system. Holding a grudge caused the

students to feel more stressed and increased their sense of discomfort over a short period.[6]

Dodie Osteen, wife of the late, great John Osteen and mother of Joel Osteen, told me years ago about how she had to forgive others as part of her supernatural healing from stage IV liver cancer, during which doctors gave her just a couple of months to live.

"I examined my heart, and God began to deal with me about some things," she wrote in her book *Healed of Cancer*. "One night I wrote letters to seven people whom I felt I might have offended, whom I needed to forgive or who needed to forgive me. I even wrote letters to people I thought I might have offended after I became sick because I had been so irritable. I hadn't been myself. One letter was to my husband; others were for each of my children and a pastor that I felt I spoke to sharply."[7]

Dodie not only defied and defeated that cancer; she has lived into her nineties and is still going strong today. Surely forgiveness was part of her healing journey.

IT'S A FACT!

A 2022 survey of two thousand adults revealed that nearly 70 percent held a grudge toward someone.[8] Bitterness impacts our physical health almost immediately. About fifteen minutes after stress hits, cortisol levels rise, and they remain elevated for hours.[9]

Some people discover that the one they have to "forgive" is God. Many people, including Christians, hold grudges against God even though He has never done anything wrong. He brings life, not death, yet people still say foolish things like, "God gave my mom cancer to teach her a lesson." That is just bad theology. God is not a child abuser. He loves us and heals us. It is Satan who steals, kills, and destroys, Jesus revealed (John 10:10).

Satan's goal is to tear us down in every area of life, but research confirms that God's antidote of forgiveness impacts our health very positively in three major areas: physical, mental, and social (relational).[10] Among people who have gone through some kind of painful conflict, a greater willingness to forgive is associated with lower blood pressure, while having forgiven someone is associated with both lower blood pressure and lower heart rate.[11]

"On the other hand," wrote Katia G. Reinert, PhD, a board-certified nurse practitioner, "a failure to forgive was associated with higher blood pressure and heart rate for longer periods of time. Failure to forgive was also associated with stress and hostility, and self-reported illness. In addition, the motivation to forgive also impacts cardiovascular risk factors....The impact of forgiveness on health can be explained by the body's response to stress. When there is perceived stress (such as in the case of feeling offended, angry or wronged) the neuro-endocrine immune mechanisms (termed allostatic stress response) are overstimulated, producing a high allostatic load. This state of chronic stress leads to impaired immunity, obesity, diabetes, and atrophy of nerve cells in the brain. However, forgiveness can protect against these effects of conflict and perceived stress....Forgiveness, it has been found, reduces the flow of cortisol."[12]

In a study of more than ten thousand Seventh-day Adventist adults who had experienced physical, emotional, or sexual abuse, neglect, and/or witnessed parental abuse before the age of eighteen, "those who scored higher in the measure of forgiving others had less negative impact of their traumatic experience on their mental health. Thus, for those adult survivors, the trait of forgiveness was protective against poor mental health."[13]

The same was true in a study of undergraduate women who experienced abuse by a boyfriend, and of men and women who went through hurtful breakups. Lack of forgiveness was associated with greater instances of depression and anxiety compared to those who more readily forgave after these types of life events.[14]

Researchers also found that readiness to forgive a spouse or friend is associated with better outcomes when resolving a betrayal and predicted greater relationship satisfaction for both the victim and the one who committed the wrong. Forgiveness brought about "increased levels of closeness, less revenge, avoidance and more benevolence towards the offender," the study found. "As a result, the offender reported increased commitment to the relationship. Therefore, forgiveness benefited both the offended and the offender....Overall, forgiveness contributes to physical, mental and social health and wellbeing not only for individuals and families, but also the community, contributing to peace and political reconciliation."[15]

THE MIND-BODY CONNECTION

I am reminded of a profound truth shared by Holocaust survivor Corrie ten Boom in her book *Tramp for the Lord*. Of her fellow concentration camp survivors she wrote: "Those who were able to forgive their former enemies were able also to return to the outside world and rebuild their lives, no matter what the physical scars. Those who nursed their bitterness remained invalids. It was as simple and as horrible as that."[16]

Two leading voices in the medical arena for forgiveness are Everett Worthington, a professor of psychology at Virginia Commonwealth University, and Loren Toussaint, a professor of psychology at Luther College, in Decorah, Iowa. "Forgiveness is a topic that's psychological, social and biological," Toussaint asserted in an article on forgiveness for *Monitor on Psychology*, a magazine published by the American Psychological Association. "It's the true mind-body connection."[17]

Bob Enright, a psychologist at the University of Wisconsin, Madison, who pioneered the study of forgiveness in the 1980s, said in the same article that "true forgiveness goes a step further, offering something positive—empathy, compassion, understanding—toward the person who hurt you. That element makes forgiveness both a virtue and a powerful construct in positive psychology."[18]

The article asserts that "forgiveness is linked to mental health outcomes such as reduced anxiety, depression and major psychiatric disorders, as well as with fewer physical health symptoms and lower mortality rates." The evidence is so substantial and compelling that Toussaint, Worthington, and fellow author/researcher David R. Williams, PhD, edited a book titled *Forgiveness and Health*, detailing all the physical and psychological benefits of forgiveness. The bottom line: "Forgiveness," Toussaint said, "allows you to let go of the chronic interpersonal stressors that cause us undue burden."[19]

IT'S A FACT!

Psychologist and forgiveness expert Bob Enright believes forgiveness can reduce or eliminate "toxic" anger. "There's nothing wrong with healthy anger," he stated, "but when anger is very deep and long lasting, it can do a number on us systemically. When you get rid of anger, your muscles relax, you're less anxious, you have more energy, your immune system can strengthen."[20]

Toussaint and his colleagues, in a study on the relationships among stress, psychological well-being, and forgiveness, found that "people who had greater levels of accumulated lifetime stress exhibited worse mental health outcomes. But among the subset of volunteers who scored high on measures of forgiveness, high lifetime stress didn't predict poor mental health. The power of forgiveness to erase that link was surprising," Toussaint said. "We thought forgiveness would knock something off the relationship [between stress and psychological distress], but we didn't expect it to zero it out."[21]

These experts agree: Anyone can become better at letting go of grudges.

"You don't have to be the world's most forgiving person," Toussaint said. "If you work at it, it takes the edge off the stress, and ultimately that helps you feel better."[22]

Let's make some positive declarations and prayers about this most important aspect of the love walk—and then we will dive deeper into the hows and whys of forgiveness with more amazing stories.

PRAYER AND DECLARATIONS

God, I commit to forgive quickly and fully. I will not hold on to bitterness and let my heart condemn me. I choose to exercise my forgiveness regularly so that forgiveness becomes part of my love nature. Only in You am I able to walk this through. Express Your mercy through my thoughts, attitudes, and actions today. Help me never to slip back into resentment. I also banish self-hatred, which has corroded and corrupted my inner life for too long. Lord, I love myself as You love me. You made me to be a carrier of Your love! I embrace my original identity in You as a fearfully and wonderfully made—and now redeemed—child of God. In Jesus' name, amen.

I will not fall into the trap of the enemy to use my conscience to condemn me. When I sense God's righteous correction, I will repent and change my behavior, walking free of the enemy's accusations.

I will not hate myself but will see myself as God sees me—as a cherished child, strong and mighty unto great works, forgiven and righteous before Him by the blood of the Lamb.

CHAPTER 8

THROW AWAY THE RECORD BOOK

ONE OF THE most profound moments of forgiveness Mary and I ever witnessed came years after our friend Jim Bakker was released from prison for crimes he did not commit. Mary and I had joined Jim Bakker and his wife in attending an outstanding Christian play at a renowned venue in Branson, Missouri. At the end of the performance, I noticed a man ten or fifteen rows in front of us waving enthusiastically to get Jim's attention.

"Jim!" this man yelled, wearing a big smile on his face. "Jim!"

I figured he was an old friend or a fan of Jim's ministry, so I said to Jim, "Look at that guy waving you down. He must really want to say hi." Jim glanced over at the man, then said, "Let's go. Let's get out of here." The man kept waving and calling, and I figured Jim hadn't really seen him or just did not want to interact with a fan.

"Jim, this guy really wants your attention," I said.

"Yeah, let's go ahead and leave," Jim repeated.

But the crowd was slow-moving, and after a while the man became impossible to ignore. Jim finally acknowledged him, and the man came up the row. They began talking, just the two of them, and as Mary and I stood there, Jim's wife told us about their history, that this man had turned his back on Jim during Jim's darkest hour. Now the two stood face to face in this auditorium at the end of a dramatic performance.

As Mary and I looked on, we recognized that something significant was happening: The man was asking Jim for forgiveness. With bated breath we wondered how Jim would respond. Then we watched as he extended his hand to the man, and they shook and clasped hands as both men began crying. The two former friends healed the gap between them in that moment.

When we got into the car, all four of us were silent. "I just need a moment," Jim said, and we honored that. That night, Jim threw away the record book of the man's misdeeds against him.

POISONOUS ROOTS IN THE BODY OF CHRIST

Bitterness between Christians seems to run deeper than the everyday kind. This is a cruel irony because the Bible emphatically tells us we must forgive and harbor no resentment, especially toward brothers and sisters in Christ. Ephesians 4:32 commands, "And be kind to one another, tenderhearted, forgiving one another, even as God in Christ forgave you." First Corinthians 13:5 says love "keeps no record of being wronged" (NLT). And Jesus said in Mark 11:25, "And whenever you stand praying, if you have anything against anyone, forgive him, that your Father in heaven may also forgive you your trespasses."

Romans 13:10 says, "Love does no wrong to one's neighbor [it never hurts anybody]. Therefore love meets all the requirements and is the fulfilling of the Law" (AMPC). In the Lord's Prayer, Jesus taught us to say, "forgive us our sins, as we have forgiven those who sin against us" (Matt. 6:12, NLT). After the Lord's Prayer, Jesus continued by saying, "For if you forgive men their trespasses, your heavenly Father will also forgive you. But if you do not forgive men their trespasses, neither will your Father forgive your trespasses" (Matt. 6:14–15).

God leaves no room for holding grudges in His kingdom. He took the record of wrongs against us and nailed it to the cross, as Paul wrote: "Having wiped out the handwriting of requirements that was against us, which was contrary to us. And He has taken it out of the way, having nailed it to the cross" (Col. 2:14). He demands that we do the same for wrongs we incur from others. We must take them to the cross and leave them there—without exceptions.

Bitterness is an especially dangerous sin because the Bible says bitterness cannot be contained. It overflows and taints others. Hebrews 12:14–15 paints the picture of bitterness as a poisonous root that will corrupt everyone around us. It says, "Work at living in peace with everyone, and work at living a holy life, for those who are not holy will not see the Lord. Look after each other so that none of you fails to receive the grace of God. Watch out that no poisonous root of bitterness grows up to trouble you, corrupting many" (NLT).

As a medical doctor I have observed that resentment is highly contagious and readily passed along like a virus. People feel justified to share their offenses, and hearers may become offended on their behalf. An offended person seems to have legitimate grief because it is heartfelt and you are only hearing their side of things. They get you to sign up for their offense, and then you are corrupted right along with them, even spreading that corruption to others.

I heard the story of a pastor who was spotted at a restaurant having lunch with a young, pretty woman. Word got around, and people grew upset, but it turned out the young woman was his granddaughter! How many people passed that story along and infected others with a wrong perception? The adage is true: One rotten apple spoils the whole barrel. And so will bitterness—and gossip—spoil the love, peace, and joy of many.

Pastors' wives seem especially prone to bitterness because they see their husbands mistreated or underappreciated. They can carry a record book with accurate details going back decades. Seeds of resentment lodge in the soil of their hearts because most of them go into ministry expecting great things and want to be loved universally. When life brings them the opposite, they are ill-equipped to respond correctly.

Other pastors and their wives, to be honest, go into ministry to be served and seen rather than to serve others. What they consider abuse and mistreatment is often the way people normally behave and is done without malice. But because it doesn't pump up their egos or raise their profiles, these wrong-headed ministers and their wives can get bent out of shape and become bitter—and that bitterness spreads fast and far.

Also, pastors invest a lot of time and energy in their congregations, and some people will leave the church over minor offenses that are usually unintentional.

But God holds no record of wrongs. Paul forgot the things that were behind him in life, including his own "church hurts," which were many and included betrayal, backbiting, and abandonment. If he had kept account of all the wrongs done to him, he would have been paralyzed with resentment.

In Luke 10:19 Jesus addressed this in a powerfully descriptive way. He said, "Behold, I give you the authority to trample on serpents and scorpions, and over all the power of the enemy, and nothing shall by any means hurt you." Are those serpents and scorpions literal? I'm sure the description includes those things, but more powerful than a snake or an insect are the demonic tormentors who bite and sting members of Christ's body so that they blame each other for their hurts! This is far more common than most people might think.

CHURCH-SPLITTING PAIN

Fred Luskin writes about a study at the University of Wisconsin, Madison, that showed a strong correlation between the amount of forgiveness people felt and their reporting of a variety of disease conditions. The more forgiving people suffered fewer illnesses. The less forgiving people reported a greater number of health problems. As Luskin writes, "This relationship held constant for both short-term physical complaints and longer-term general well-being....The relationship between forgiveness and health held true for the frequency of symptoms reported. People who had a higher capacity for forgiveness reported fewer symptoms than those with a less developed ability to forgive. People with higher capacities for forgiveness also reported fewer medically diagnosed chronic conditions. This study established a fundamental relationship between learning to forgive and reported incidences of health complaints."[1]

LETTING GO OF THE "ANGRY LIST"

A patient in her midseventies came into my office with her husband six months ago. She had fibromyalgia, and chronic pain was robbing her of sleep. Her muscles were tense, and her whole back was contracted. Tight muscles constrict blood vessels, sometimes causing ischemia so that metabolic waste products can't get out and oxygen and fresh blood can't get in, which causes pain. What happens when you clench your fist for just a few minutes? It starts aching pretty fast. Now imagine that happening all over your body for most of the day.

I checked this woman for deadly emotions and found she was plagued by unforgiveness.

"Who are you angry at?" I asked her.

"My church split, and half the church left," she said. "I'm angry at the pastor and other leaders who took a lot of the members."

I asked her how many people she thought she was angry at, and she came up with a list of thirty! No wonder her muscles were so bound up. She was in fight mode all the time against this group of people—at least in her own mind.

"You signed up for fibromyalgia," I informed her. "Do you want to hold on to it or get rid of it?"

Her husband chimed in, "I've told her to release it. She just won't. She thinks she has some right to carry this resentment around forever."

"Do you want to get better or not?" I asked her. "Is it worth it to go through life like you have been doing, with all these physical problems manifesting?"

"No, I want to get rid of this pain!" she cried. "I have not slept well for ten or fifteen years. I'm taking all these meds. I feel dopey and strange, like I'm not living. I feel horrible! I will do whatever it takes."

With her input, I wrote out the name of every person she had not forgiven. Then I had her speak what the Word says about forgiveness.

"Forgive with your heart, not your head, according to Ephesians 4:32," I instructed her.

We worked through the list, naming each person and having her forgive them by name, sincerely and from her heart. Her husband sat there looking at me like, "This doctor is crazy. This will never work."

But the effect was amazing. The woman's whole body relaxed. All the pain and stress went away. Now when I verbalized the names of most of these past "offenders," she had no stress or tension response. On a couple of names she still tightened up, so we had to forgive them again with the heart instead of the mind. The peace of God came upon her. She broke out in laughter. You could see the joy of God on her face in the absence of the emotional garbage she had kept locked up inside her.

Forgiving worked better and much faster than any of the medical interventions she had undergone for more than a decade. Kenneth Hagin Sr. wrote something amazing about forgiveness and disease in his book *Love: The Way to Victory*: "For more than sixty years in the ministry, I have said that if my faith didn't work and my prayers weren't answered, unforgiveness is the first place I would look. I'm not saying that all sickness and disease is caused by unforgiveness. I'm just saying that's the first place I would look."[2]

Hagin recounted how person after person had told him the same thing—they had to forgive someone before they could receive their healing. Some of them were even terminal cases. "One man told me, 'My doctor said, "You'll be dead in thirty days."' The man just made the necessary adjustments in his heart by getting rid of every bit of ill will, animosity, and unforgiveness, and he's healed and still alive today. I never did have to pray for him or lay hands on him. Think about that—he was healed of terminal cancer when he exercised forgiveness!"[3]

DEAL GENTLY WITH OTHERS

We cannot just forgive people flippantly and move on. Part of the love walk is being tender with each other. As Ephesians 4:30–32 says (emphasis added),

> And do not grieve the Holy Spirit of God, by whom you were sealed for the day of redemption. Let all bitterness, wrath, anger, clamor, and evil speaking be put away from you, with all malice. And *be kind to one another, tender-hearted, forgiving one another, even as God in Christ forgave you.*

Kindness is an important element of forgiveness. Jim Bakker could have forgiven the man who turned his back on him when he was in prison without any expression of affection or acceptance, but that is just not the way God expects it to be done. Scientific research tells us of the physical benefits of kindness.

"When people feel securely attached, their stress levels go down," Dr. Helen Riess, director of the Empathy and Relational Science Program at Massachusetts General Hospital, told *Time* magazine. "Just being in the presence of someone who greets us with positive regard and caring can actually lower those levels of cortisol and adrenaline and create greater homeostasis, which means that your neurochemicals are back in balance."[4]

The problem is that far more people think society is growing ruder, not kinder, according to a Statista survey.[5] Whatever the reasons for this, rudeness and harshness can get in the way of our expression of forgiveness and affect—even ruin—our attempts to foster reconciliation when appropriate. In 1 Corinthians 5:1–5 (NLT) Paul illuminated a troubling situation in the Corinthian church that many of us would rightly consider outrageous. He wrote:

I can hardly believe the report about the sexual immorality going on among you—something that even pagans don't do. I am told that a man in your church is living in sin with his stepmother. You are so proud of yourselves, but you should be mourning in sorrow and shame. And you should remove this man from your fellowship. Even though I am not with you in person, I am with you in the Spirit. And as though I were there, I have already passed judgment on this man in the name of the Lord Jesus. You must call a meeting of the church. I will be present with you in spirit, and so will the power of our Lord Jesus. Then you must throw this man out and hand him over to Satan so that his sinful nature will be destroyed and he himself will be saved on the day the Lord returns.

Paul handed this man over to Satan for his own sake and the church's. Most of us would consider that a strong response, but in his next letter to the Corinthian believers, Paul counseled the gentle restoration of this same man. He wrote, "I am not overstating it when I say that the man who caused all the trouble hurt all of you more than he hurt me. Most of you opposed him, and that was punishment enough. Now, however, it is time to forgive and comfort him. Otherwise he may be overcome by discouragement. So I urge you now to reaffirm your love for him" (2 Cor. 2:5–8, NLT).

Wow! This man had engaged in seriously immoral, damaging behavior, yet Paul considered it important that he be restored when he repented. Why? Because Paul knew that divisions within the body become the biggest openings for tormentors to enter.

I wrote to you as I did to test you and see if you would fully comply with my instructions. When you forgive this man, I forgive him, too. And when I forgive whatever needs to be forgiven, I do so with Christ's authority for your benefit, *so that Satan will not outsmart us. For we are familiar with his evil schemes.*

—2 CORINTHIANS 2:9–11, NLT, EMPHASIS ADDED

Forgiving people is directly connected to avoiding and defeating Satan's "evil schemes" so he "will not outsmart us." Unforgiveness gives the devil open access to our lives. If we do not forgive, comfort, reaffirm our love, and gently restore to fellowship people who have sinned, we give Satan an open door.

Jesus displayed this same merciful approach to the woman caught in adultery.

As he was speaking, the teachers of religious law and the Pharisees brought a woman who had been caught in the act of adultery. They put her in front of the crowd. "Teacher," they said to Jesus, "this woman was caught in the act of adultery. The law of Moses says to stone her. What do you say?" They were trying to trap him into saying something they could use against him, but Jesus stooped down and wrote in the dust with his finger. They kept demanding an answer, so he stood up again and said, "All right, but let the one who has never sinned throw the first stone!" Then he stooped down again and wrote in the dust. When the accusers heard this, they slipped away one by one, beginning with the oldest, until only Jesus was left in the middle of the crowd with the woman. Then Jesus stood up again and said to the woman, "Where are your accusers? Didn't even one of them condemn you?" "No, Lord," she said. And Jesus said, "Neither do I. Go and sin no more."

—JOHN 8:3–11, NLT

Even to Christian readers Jesus' way of handling this sinful woman can seem outrageous. Where is the punishment? The admonishment? The stern rebuke? Yet Jesus knew what we do not—the heart of this woman and the exact situation which had brought her before Him. His approach was gentle, tender, while not compromising on sin. We too should work to restore and reaffirm our love for people who have committed even egregious wrongs so the devil has no room to work his schemes.

One longitudinal study on female nurses examined forgiveness, health, and well-being in midlife. "Results showed that forgiveness was significantly associated with better psychosocial well-being outcomes such as...social integration and decreased psychological distress outcomes such as depressive symptoms. It concluded that forgiveness may have population mental health implications in promoting psychosocial well-being."[6]

What that means in plain terms is that forgiveness builds up communities, while bitterness tears them down.

SUPERNATURAL MEDICINE

Love expressing itself through forgiveness and much more is so powerful that I knew I needed to make it a central part of my medical practice, not just some side suggestion. I had always checked people to see if they were getting the proper nutrients, eating the right diet, engaging in good exercise appropriate to their age and condition, and treating any diseases or conditions they might have. Now I added spiritual checks and prescriptions to my assessments and prognoses. I asked about their relationships, their emotions, and their spirituality. In addition to giving clinical treatments, I invited the presence and work of the Holy Spirit, and I prescribed prayer, confession of the

Word of God, forgiveness, and other behaviors that put love into action.

IT'S A FACT!

Forgiveness enhances our immune functioning. Participants in one study who were more forgiving also had measurably stronger immune systems compared to those who were less willing to forgive.[7] Medical research tells us that as much as 80 percent of illness and disease is related to stress.[8] Holding on to grudges opens the door for diseases to secure a foothold in our bodies. Chronic stress also speeds up the development of cancerous tumors.[9]

One of the most effective things I do for my patients is what I have done for myself for years: I give them powerful sermons to watch or listen to. Some readers might roll their eyes at the idea of giving a sermon, podcast, or teaching video as part of a health prescription, but good Bible-based, Spirit-inspired preaching and teaching is literally life to us. Paul said we must teach and admonish one another with all wisdom. Jesus said His words are spirit and life (John 6:63). Proverbs 18:21 says death and life are in the power of the tongue. Peter said we speak to each other "as the oracles of God" (1 Pet. 4:11).

Those are amazing spiritual truths! Clicking on an internet video or tapping on a podcast is much more than seeking a few hours of diversion or learning; it's administering supernatural medicine to your whole being through inspired words of Scripture and Bible-based teaching. What we listen to or watch is not a casual thing! Everything either gives life or produces death, and even if something seems to do neither, it uses up your time. Good, biblical teaching is literally like a dose of medicine.

I treated a woman recently and helped her to forgive herself. I also wrote her a prescription, part of which was to say three times a day, "I forgive myself, I accept myself, and I love myself." She had not felt love for herself in thirty years, so a pill was not going to help her. You should have seen the glow on her face! This woman had come in appearing sick from a steep decline in her kidney function, which was taking her quickly toward dialysis. Now in place of the spirit of death and heaviness was a light in her eyes, a newfound joy in her face, and a sense of optimism and love that can only come from the presence of God resting on you. The transformation, which happened within minutes, was absolutely amazing.

To keep the healing happening, I prescribed powerful confessions based on God's Word and several powerful sermons for her to watch daily as part of maintaining her overall health. When prescribing teachings, I always incline my ear to the Holy Spirit and listen to which preacher and message He may indicate to me. He often guides my mind and heart to the right one.

In addition to this, there are a number of ways we can become more forgiving toward people. Some involve formal strategies that have been tested by those who spend their careers studying forgiveness.

Enright, the expert referenced earlier, created a twenty-step forgiveness process model to move people through four phases: uncovering one's negative feelings about the offense, deciding to forgive, working toward understanding the offending person, and discovering empathy and compassion for him or her. "Enright has shown this model is effective in various one-on-one interventions, including a study that showed it alleviated depression, anxiety and PTSD in women who have experienced spousal emotional abuse," according to one article.[10] Enright is quoted as saying, "Through these cognitive exercises, they begin to see the other person [the offender] as a wounded human being, as opposed to stereotyping them and defining them by their hurtful actions."[11]

Worthington developed what he calls the REACH Forgiveness model, a five-step process that also emphasizes finding empathy for the person who hurt them and persisting in a posture of forgiveness over the long haul. His model is often employed in group settings.

In a meta-analysis of fifty-four forgiveness studies, Worthington found that both his and Enright's models helped people forgive and also improved their mental health, according to a review. "There's a strong dose-response relationship between the amount of time people try to forgive and the amount of forgiveness they're successful at experiencing. It's all about the time spent," Worthington said. "You run people through a six-hour group, not only do they forgive but they also reduce their levels of depression and anxiety."[12]

Toussaint has observed that many people stop short of the goal and conclude they are naturally bitter people. His words are gold: "A natural resurgence of unforgiving feelings is normal. It's like having a piece of cake during a diet. Just because you have a setback doesn't mean you're an unforgiving person."[13]

Some people give up because they believe forgiveness means making oneself vulnerable to the same pain again or abandoning any possibility of receiving justice. But forgiveness and justice are two separate topics, and most of us know by now that forgiveness does not require reconciliation. While we may forgive someone, we are not required in every situation to establish a new, close relationship with him or her. As Worthington explained, "Whether I forgive or don't forgive isn't going to affect whether justice is done....Forgiveness happens inside my skin."[14]

Neither is letting go of offenses a sign of weakness. Jesus, the Creator of the universe and the omnipotent God, says mercy and forgiveness are part of His eternal character. In other words, forgiving others is among the strongest things you can do.

Let me make a bold statement: We as doctors have missed the most powerful key to living a long, healthy, prosperous life. It is simply walking in love and forgiveness toward one another. Love is the key to becoming disease-resistant. The good news is that you don't need to come into my office to have me take you through the steps of forgiveness. You can lift up heartfelt, life-changing prayer right where you sit and destroy strongholds of bitterness and hatred just as I do when I take people through forgiveness therapy. Take your Bible and open it to Ephesians 4:32. Let's pray and declare these truths together.

PRAYER AND DECLARATIONS

God, I commit without reservation to forgive others as Christ has forgiven me. That is impossible in my own strength, but I am not relying on my own strength; I am relying on Yours. Please look into the areas of pain in my heart—the places I don't want to think about or even acknowledge where people or situations have hurt me deeply. I yield these places completely to You. Nail them to the cross! I no longer own those situations because they have been placed under Your blood.

Thank You for forgiving me in the many ways I have hurt others, even when I've been unaware of it. Help them to forgive me as I forgive those who hurt me. Lord, You never hold on to bitterness or resentment. You always refrain from reacting wrongly, and over time You work to restore us gently, even when we have betrayed You. Help me to be like You! Shape my character so it comes more easily to forgive than to condemn and seek revenge. Amen.

I declare that I don't want bad things to befall people who have hurt me. I let go of any desired outcome for revenge, and I trust God to deal justly, mercifully, and gently with people who have hurt or opposed me or my loved ones.

My life will be characterized by mercy and quick forgiveness, no longer by wells of poisonous pain and being stuck in the past. I am a new creation in Christ, and I willingly lose all capacity to recall offenses and rehearse wrongs done to me. The fragrance of forgiveness is upon my life.

At one time I held on to bitterness toward these people: [name them]. But I now release and cancel the debt of each one of them from any apology they owe to me. I release [name them again, one by one] from anything they did to me or my loved ones.

By setting these people free, I liberate myself from the poison of bitterness. I will no longer allow corruption to spread through my life via the power of bitterness.

As God no longer remembers my sins and iniquities (Heb. 10:17), I practice divine forgetfulness and forgive and forget all wrongs done to me, and I will keep no record of wrongs (1 Cor. 13:5, NIV).

I am at peace and at rest as I look to the future free of unforgiveness or others' unpaid debts toward me. In allowing them to walk free and clear, I clear the way for my own future to be blessed, peaceful, joyful, and more loving and forgiving than I ever dreamed.

The love commandment also involves loving yourself and not allowing others to repeatedly abuse and hurt you. You must establish boundaries to protect yourself, and remember that some people need to be loved from a distance.

SECTION III:
OVERCOMING PESSIMISM

CHAPTER 9

THE CAUSES OF HOPELESSNESS

ALONG WITH MANY others in the medical profession, I believe America is experiencing an epidemic of depression, and the resulting plague of pessimism is affecting the old as well as the young. Studies show that depression and pessimism are related and mutually reinforcing. A pessimistic attitude among people who are not depressed actually predicts who will become depressed and stay depressed. Choosing optimism—another way of saying we embrace God's hope-filled perspective on our lives—actually relieves depression.[1]

Pessimism acts as a silent infiltrator. It creeps in almost unnoticed over time. Nobody stands up one day and announces, "I'm going to be a pessimist from here forward!" But after experiencing a few of life's adverse events and being buffeted by bad news, people can slip into the grip of this negative mindset. They view events, people, and circumstances in a hopeless way, with little or no expectation that things will improve. The Survey Center on American Life found that 53 percent of Americans are either very or somewhat pessimistic. This tendency toward pessimism seems to increase as people get older. Think about it—over half the population of America expects the worst to happen and automatically assumes that bad outcomes are inevitable. That is an epidemic by any standard.[2]

A hopeless paradigm pervades the church as well. In my observation, many pastors and people in the pews are just as pessimistic as non-Christians are. While they should be flourishing in the love walk and demonstrating the overcoming power of God's love to a watching world, their hope is paralyzed by thinking that tells them, "This is the way things are, and they will never get better." They quit expecting God to come through for them; they stop believing in His miracle-working power. They lose their joy and peace because they think they can't rely on His protection or provision. The light of Christ within them grows dim because their hope is extinguished bit by bit.

The root cause of pessimism is usually some type of trauma—an accident, divorce, failed relationship, loss of a loved one, loss of a pet, financial distress, physical injury or illness, and so on. Pessimism can also be instilled by a parent, teacher, coach, or anyone in authority who inculcates this viewpoint into young minds. For some, the steady drumbeat of hurts and everyday disappointments drives them to become pessimistic because it seems easier to expect the worst than to expose themselves to renewed pain from dashed hopes.

Pessimists anchor themselves to disbelief and suspicion instead of faith, hope, and love. Even when things seem to be going well for them or others, they set the radio dial in their minds to their preferred preset and say, "Things are bound to get worse at some point," or, "Good times never last." In doing so, they literally prophesy their future and program themselves to fail. Pessimism is a meditation on failure rather than hope, and what we meditate on gives birth to results, usually through our own actions or inaction. Pessimists therefore make plans to miss the mark.

Even secular social scientists recognize that pessimism and optimism are both self-fulfilling. One leading researcher of "learned optimism," psychologist Martin Seligman, says that after twenty-five years of research he is convinced a pessimistic outlook—believing that misfortune is not only our fault but long lasting and capable of ruining our efforts—makes us more prone to experiencing such misfortune. This can lead to depression, lower achievements, and even physical illness.[3]

If a non-Christian academic researcher can observe the real-life effects of hopelessness, how much more should Christians recognize and address them!

LEARNING TO HOPE

The good news is that God is full of hope, and He expects His children to be hopeful too. It's our birthright and a vital aspect of the love walk. God is not pessimistic in any way, and He did not design us to be pessimistic. There is no such thing as a "pessimistic personality" or a "negative person" except by choice. Seligman's groundbreaking book *Learned Optimism* overturned ideas about pessimism's causes and cures. In it, he writes:

> A pessimistic attitude may seem so deeply rooted as to be permanent. I have found, however, that *pessimism is escapable. Pessimists can in fact learn to be optimists,* and not through mindless devices like whistling a happy tune or mouthing platitudes ("Every day, in every way, I'm getting better and better"), but by learning a new set of cognitive skills.[4]

Seligman and others have come to the same conclusions the Bible has offered for thousands of years: God did not make anyone to be a pessimist. Therefore, pessimism is not a permanent condition unless you choose to make it so. Godly, faith-filled thinking—secular experts call it optimism—can be chosen and indeed must be chosen for individuals to lead the satisfying, successful lives God has planned for them. As Seligman concluded, thinking habits aren't permanent. People can choose how they think. Unlike other personal traits, pessimism isn't fixed and can be changed. By learning specific skills, one can break free from pessimism and embrace optimism when desired.[5]

This is fantastic news for our health because higher levels of hope have been shown to help people deal successfully with pain and some forms of illness.[6] Optimistic people live longer and have fewer illnesses.[7]

In an eleven-year study, the authors investigated the connection between optimism, pessimism, and patients suffering with coronary heart disease. Levels of optimism and pessimism were determined using a standardized test. Eleven years later, those results and follow-up data about coronary heart disease as a cause of death were used to calculate odds, with adjustments made for cardiovascular disease risk. The study found, amazingly or perhaps predictably, that those who died because of coronary heart disease "were significantly more pessimistic at baseline than the others. This finding applies to both men and women.

Among the study subjects in the highest quartile of pessimism, the adjusted risk of death caused by coronary heart disease was approximately 2.2-fold compared to the subjects in the lowest quartile." The authors concluded that "pessimism seems to be a substantial risk factor for death from CHD [coronary heart disease]. As an easily measured variable, it might be a very useful tool together with the other known risk factors to determine the risk of CHD-induced mortality."[8]

In their book *The Biology of Kindness*, Immaculata De Vivo and Daniel Lumera cited a 2019 review published in JAMA Network Open by Alan Rozanski, a cardiologist at Mount Sinai Morningside hospital in New York City. Rozanski compared the results of fifteen studies for a total of 229,391 participants and found that those with higher levels of optimism experienced a 35 percent lower risk of cardiovascular events compared to those with lower optimism, as well as a lower mortality rate.[9]

They also presented research led by Lewina Lee at Harvard University analyzing 69,744 women from the NHS and 1,429 men from the aging study of the US Department of Veterans Affairs. "The results tell us that optimists tend to live on average 11 to 15 percent longer than pessimists and have an excellent chance of achieving 'exceptional longevity'—that is, by definition, an age of over 85 years."[10]

Studies also show that spiritually minded people cope better with loss and illness.[11] Depression is a risk factor for heart disease and may predict who will leave the hospital alive after a heart attack.[12] And a recent study showed that depressed people are at significantly greater risk of a stroke.[13]

Hope results in longer and healthier lives, but to realize these benefits we must learn how to root out pessimism.

IT'S A FACT!

Among women facing breast cancer for a second time, the ones who survive longer are those who express "great joy in living" and choose optimism.[14]

EXPLANATORY STYLE

Each one of us keeps an ongoing internal dialogue on what we see and perceive. We essentially explain reality to ourselves, and leading thinkers in psychology and counseling call this our explanatory style. Everybody has one. It is the way we make sense of the world and come to conclusions about why events happen and what eventual outcomes are likely to be.

The pessimist is stuck in a negative explanatory style, while optimists see difficult circumstances with a more hopeful outlook. As Seligman puts it, the way you interpret events affects whether you feel helpless or motivated when facing everyday challenges or major setbacks. This explanatory style is akin to carrying a guiding word in your heart—either a "no" or a "yes"—which shapes your attitude toward life.[15]

In biblical terms, optimists are open to hopeful explanations, while pessimists reject them. Jesus told a parable that speaks to this profoundly. In the familiar account, a sower went out to sow seed, "And it came to pass, as he sowed, some fell by the way side, and the fowls of the air came and devoured it up" (Mark 4:4, KJV). Those seeds represent the gospel message, and hope is a big part of the gospel—hope that God cares for us and loves us and has a good future for each one of us.

The "wayside" Jesus spoke of was hard-beaten ground, soil so frequently tread upon that it had become a path or road. Pessimism is one form of hard soil. It actively resists any hopeful thought or influence. Pessimistic thinking makes it almost impossible to plant seeds of hope or any other godly belief in one's heart. It rejects God's view of the future and instead opts to believe that there is no hope ahead. The "birds" in the parable are Satan and his demons, who take those seeds of hope and life away when we reject them. So the pessimist lives the self-fulfilling prophecy of rejecting hope, then living in the resulting gloom and misery.

Pessimism, like worry, fear, and doubt, is a fleshly mindset promoted by Satan. Earlier I called pessimism a "preset," and Romans 8:5 uses similar language, saying, "For those who live according to the flesh set their minds on the things of the flesh, but those who live according to the Spirit, the things of the Spirit."

"Setting our minds" on one belief or another is the same as saying it is our explanatory style. Disappointments, adversity, illness, accidents, relationship problems, loss of a job, and other stressful events eventually occur in all our lives—but we have the choice to interpret these to ourselves in a hopeful, God-honoring way or a negative, pessimistic way. Each ungodly preset invites deadly emotions into our minds and bodies, which destroy our faith, rob us of peace and joy (and all the other fruits of the Spirit; see Galatians 5:22–23), and eventually contribute to disease and an early death.

Seligman asserts that how you interpret negative events, or your explanatory style, goes beyond the words you use when you mess up. It's a mindset formed during childhood and adolescence and is shaped by how you perceive your role in the world—whether as someone who is worthy and capable or one who is unworthy and hopeless. Your explanatory style ultimately determines whether you are an optimist or a pessimist.[16]

Let's look at the elements of a pessimistic explanatory style.

THE BLAMERS: "IT'S PERSONAL"

Three key aspects define a pessimist's explanatory style: personalization, permanence, and pervasiveness.

Pessimists personalize everything. They blame themselves for hurtful events and accept the pain of regret as their just reward. They agree with Satan, whom the Bible calls the accuser—the blamer—of the brethren (Rev. 12:10). When something painful happens, they say, "It's all my fault. I failed somehow. I am to blame." As a result, they see themselves as helpless and contemptible.

"People who blame themselves when they fail have low self-esteem as a consequence," Seligman tells us. "They think they are worthless, talentless, and unlovable." On the other hand, "People who blame external events do not lose self-esteem when bad events strike. On the whole, they like themselves better than people who blame themselves do."[17]

It's irrational to think we are responsible for negative external events we did not cause, and yet pessimists default to that position.

FAILURE MENTALITY: "IT'S PERVASIVE"

Pessimists don't limit the scope of their hopelessness but expand it to encompass all circumstances at all times. They "catastrophize" by expecting the worst outcomes in all situations because they believe bad outcomes and failure are normal—even unavoidable. In this way their pessimism becomes virtually a religion. To them, it explains everything and predicts everything.

For example, a young man goes on multiple dates and is repeatedly rejected. Finally he concludes that all women dislike him and he will never find a wife. This conclusion combines personalization and pervasiveness, and we hear this kind of sentiment in many forms. A person with a pessimistic outlook makes universal explanations such as the following:

"All men are cheaters."

"All police officers are against me."

"I am unattractive to all men."

"I come into conflict with every boss I have."

Each of these statements is an example of practicing faith in reverse. In Mark 11:24 (KJV) Jesus said, "Therefore I say unto you, what things soever ye desire, when ye pray, believe that ye receive them, and ye shall have them." The pessimist believes the opposite: that whatever he or she desires, he or she shall not have. They employ faith in exactly the wrong direction and become so negative and sour in the process that their predictions become self-fulfilling prophecies. Who wants to marry a negative, downcast person except maybe another negative, downcast person?

Optimists—that is, hopeful people—do the opposite when bad things happen. They believe difficulties are limited in scope and duration, arise from specific causes, and are abnormal, giving way to an inevitable future full of good things.[18]

Instead of saying, "I am unattractive to all men," they say, "I may be unattractive to some men, but most men think I am attractive."

A pessimistic mindset indeed proves to be pervasive and will undermine every aspect of a person's success and satisfaction. It leads them to seek control and predictability by making universal explanations to try to understand and brace themselves for negative outcomes. People who fall into pessimistic, pervasive thinking believe that a failure in one area of life will spill over and affect all other aspects of their lives. When they add personalization to this, then everything becomes their fault. The bitterness of life, in their eyes, becomes deeply personal and beyond their control. They believe nothing will work out for them and that one unfortunate event will ruin their entire lives.

PERMANENT THINKING: "NEVER" AND "ALWAYS"

Pessimists explain negative events to themselves using words like *never* and *always*. For instance, "I never get good breaks. The worst thing always happens to me." This is the basis for the toxic bit of worldly wisdom people call "Murphy's Law"—the idea that the worst outcome is inevitable. That is not a law at all but what the Bible calls an evil foreboding (Prov. 15:15, AMPC). It does not come from the heart of God and is not part of the love walk.

On the other side, optimistic people explain good events to themselves in terms of permanent causes: "Something good always comes up. Love always finds a way." Oral Roberts would say every week on his national TV program, "Something good is going to happen to you." The optimist attributes good things to their own traits and abilities, while pessimists credit good things to transient, unpredictable causes outside of themselves.[19]

IT'S A FACT!

"Your explanatory style stems directly from your view of your place in the world—whether you think you are valuable and deserving, or worthless and hopeless. It is the hallmark of whether you are an optimist or a pessimist."[20]

"Optimists recover from [failure] immediately," Seligman writes. "Very soon after failing, they pick themselves up, shrug, and start trying again. For them, defeat is a challenge, a mere setback on the road to inevitable victory....Pessimists wallow in defeat, which they see as permanent and pervasive."[21]

Research has also found that people who resist pessimistic thinking view the causes of negative events as temporary. If you often describe bad situations using words like "always" and "never," or attribute them to fixed traits, you have a persistent, pessimistic mindset, according to Seligman. However, if you use terms such as "sometimes" and "recently" and blame bad events on temporary factors, you have an optimistic outlook.[22]

Pessimistic "never" and "always" language sounds like this:

"I will always be broke."

"I will never get out of this rut."

"I will never find my life mate."

"I won't ever find a good job."

"This bad situation will go on forever."

Mother Teresa had no patience for pessimists or any form of complaining. "Another seemingly minor fault that occupied a prominent place in Mother Teresa's list of 'significant' sins was grumbling," one account of her life reads. "For her, grumbling pointed to a lack of practical faith, to the failure to see God's hand in the particular circumstances, to reluctance to surrender to His will." Mother Teresa also considered moodiness a type of "sickness" and placed it on "the list of spiritual ailments that seriously hinder love. Moodiness, a form of passive retaliation, manifested by stubbornly and silently showing one's dissatisfaction, revealed the inner reality of many hidden sins: pride, anger, lack of forgiveness, resentment. Moodiness has a paralyzing effect on others (community or family), but even more so on the one who gives into this fault, as it cripples his or her ability to love and grow in love. If joy is contagious, so is the lack of it."[23]

Optimists, by contrast, choose to focus on the good in life instead of dwelling on the bad. They compartmentalize and contain negative events while letting hope rule their thoughts and emotions. If they use "always" and "never," it is on the positive side.

RECEIVING CORRECTION

So many Christians are mired in pessimism that for their own good they need to recognize it, repent, and return to the love walk before negativity destroys their lives. Sometimes to get back into the flow of God's love we must be jolted into it by a word of correction. This happened to me in my own love revolution, which I shared about earlier. Jesus often startled His hearers with a word of rebuke or by reframing a question such as, "Where is your faith?" (Luke 8:25).

Staying in the love walk involves receiving life-giving correction lest we drift away without realizing it. I am reminded of the Korean Airlines flight on September 1, 1983, that had flown from New York City to Anchorage, Alaska, and the second leg of the flight from Anchorage to Seoul, South Korea. It went off course and ended up in Soviet (Russian) airspace. The aircraft was shot down, and all 269 passengers on board lost their lives. Why did it go off course in the first place? The pilot failed to engage the autopilot, allowing it to depart from its intended course. At first the variation was small, but over time it grew so large that the airplane was shot down by a Soviet fighter jet. A small amount of correction early on could have saved the plane from being miles away from where it intended to be.[24]

Love will correct us, but love will never punish us. Proverbs 3:11–12 says, "My son, do not despise the chastening of the LORD, nor detest His correction; for whom the LORD loves He corrects."

The writer of Hebrews considered this such an important principle that he quoted it in his own letter (Heb. 12:5–6).

Most Christians I have worked with do not take correction well at all. They whine, murmur, and complain. I hear this blame-shifting daily in my practice when meeting with Christian patients of all different kinds. Instead of welcoming suggestions to correct their courses, they find or create another culprit—anything to exonerate themselves. It should come as no surprise that those who resist correction are those who drift furthest from the love walk. They are unwilling to receive the life-giving rebukes of the Lord.

Take a moment to ask yourself, "Do I recognize my own attitudes and behavior in the descriptions of pessimists above? Do I expect the worst, catastrophize difficult events, default to a hopeless attitude, blame myself, take failure personally, and expect most things to go wrong?" If so, you need to repent and get back onto the love walk. God has something much better for you, and it begins by rediscovering hope.

Nobody is ever "too far gone" or too negative to return to the path of life. Seligman, an expert in this field of study, wrote, "The good news is that pessimists can learn the skills of optimism and permanently improve the quality of their lives."[25] Those skills, which will free you from the prison of pessimistic thinking, are the subject of the next chapter.

Note: If you are struggling with pessimism, consider finding a Christian counselor or psychologist who practices cognitive behavioral therapy.

Prayer and Declarations

Lord, I repent of any vestige of pessimism I have allowed to infect and dominate my thoughts and emotions. Please forgive me. I confess the areas where I have lost hope [speak those specific areas]. You have not lost hope. You do not see me as a failure or permanently messed-up. You have a glorious future planned for me! Free me from the tendency to think in personal, pervasive, and permanent ways about difficult circumstances. I commit myself to return fully to the love walk with my hope restored, growing more optimistic and more in love with You each day. Amen.

I renounce any hopeless thought as being from the devil, not from God.

I declare that I am a hopeful person. Hope is my inheritance.

I refuse to give the enemy more credit than he is due. When hard things happen, I proclaim that they are limited in duration and scope—they are "light and momentary" and soon will pass.

There is nothing self-protective or wise about being pessimistic or expecting the worst. Rather, great power is in our hope when our hope is in God.

I serve the "God of all hope," and His hope is my hope as I stay in the love walk.

I repent for being a long-term blamer of myself when I did not meet my expectations. I boldly confess that I am worthy, I am talented, and I am lovable.

A perceived failure in one area of my life will not spill over and affect all aspects of my life, because Philippians 4:13 says, "I can do all things through Christ who strengthens me."

I refuse to explain negative events using "never" and "always," implying that the negative event will always occur, but I boldly confess that something good is going to happen to me every day!

CHAPTER 10

DEVELOPING UNSHAKABLE HOPE

PSYCHOLOGIST MARTIN SELIGMAN conducted a well-known study in 1990 involving competitive college swimmers. In it, coaches asked their athletes to swim as best they could during a competition, and then the swimmers were given false results that disappointed them. After a couple of hours of rest, the swimmers swam a second race, "and the results between the optimists and pessimists were significantly different. The pessimists were on average 1.6 percent slower than during their first performance, while the optimists swam 0.5 percent faster." The interpretation of the experiment was that optimists tend to use failure as a goal to do better, whereas pessimists tend to be discouraged more easily and give up more readily.[1]

Optimism and pessimism also empirically affect how our cells age. In 2012, researchers Elizabeth Blackburn and Elissa Epel "identified a correlation between pessimism and accelerated telomere shortening in a group of postmenopausal women," wrote authors Immaculata De Vivo and Daniel Lumera in *The Biology of Kindness*. Telomeres, according to the National Library of Medicine, "are protein structures located at the ends of each eukaryotic DNA chromosomal arm" that "play a significant role in cellular senescence [decay] with major contributions to human aging."[2]

Blackburn and Epel's study found that a pessimistic attitude may be associated with shorter telomeres. In plain English, that means a negative outlook on life can literally affect how quickly our cells—meaning our entire bodies—age.

In 2021, scientists from Harvard University, Boston University, and the Ospedale Maggiore in Milan carefully examined the telomeres of 490 elderly men in the Normative Health Study on US veterans. "Subjects with strongly pessimistic attitudes were associated with shorter telomeres—a further encouraging finding in the study of those mechanisms that make optimism and pessimism biologically relevant."[3]

While science lauds the health benefits of optimism and what the Bible calls "hope," the very meaning of hope seems to have been watered down over time, even among Christians. We almost use it as a fond but unrealistic notion, a faint wish for a good outcome, something from *The Wizard of Oz* or a song sung by a Disney fairy godmother. But biblical hope is one of the strongest forces in existence. It is a powerful expectancy, a fully convinced desire for some positive result. It is an anticipation that leads to action, a life-giving attitude, and an energizing hunger for an excellent outcome.

Hope is an expectation, not a wish upon a star. It's like expecting a baby. You know it's in there; you have no doubt about it, though you have not seen it with your own eyes yet.

You can't have faith without hope, and you can't have hope without expectation. Most pessimists have lost their hope and expectation and are expecting the worst things to happen in their life. Jerry Savelle was a man of great faith and great hope and great expectation. He walked in the favor of God every day, and he confessed favor over his life every day. Jerry said that the more he acknowledged favor, the more he expected favor, and the more he expected favor, the more he experienced favor.

Love, hope, and faith are close companions. Members of this trio are often mentioned together in Scripture, such as in Paul's famous "love chapter" of 1 Corinthians 13, where he wrote, "And now abide faith, hope, love, these three; but the greatest of these is love" (v. 13). In Romans he wrote, "Now hope does not disappoint, because the love of God has been poured out in our hearts by the Holy Spirit who was given to us" (5:5). Love and hope together create great confidence for good outcomes. As Paul wrote, love "believes all things, hopes all things, endures all things" (1 Cor. 13:7).

Hope is the antithesis and perfect antidote to pessimism. The two attitudes cannot coexist. We choose to let one or the other dominate our minds. To be a successful Christian and overcome pessimism, we must walk in all three: hope, faith, and love. They mutually reinforce one another like a threefold cord, which is not quickly broken (Eccles. 4:12).

How Hope Affects Health

Hope, like all the attributes of God, results in many health benefits, including the following:

- Lower rates of depression
- Better psychological and physical well-being
- Greater resistance to depression
- Lower levels of pain and distress

Hopeful people are:

- Better able to handle stress
- More likely to exercise
- More likely to follow a healthy diet
- More likely to live with a spouse
- Less likely to smoke
- More likely to follow medical advice

Optimists live as much as 15 percent longer than pessimists, live happier lives than pessimists, are more successful than pessimists, and are more likely to achieve their life goals than pessimists.

Optimism and pessimism, Seligman found, directly impact health, almost as much as physical factors. Optimists contract fewer infections and maintain better health habits compared to pessimists. Optimism may also boost the immune system, and research indicates that optimists may live longer than pessimists.[4]

In a British study, sixty-nine women with breast cancer were followed for five years. Those patients who had what Seligman called a "fighting spirit" were more likely to avoid a recurrence of the disease, while those who either died or experienced a relapse tended to view their initial diagnosis with helplessness and passive acceptance.[5]

In a later study of thirty-four women facing breast cancer for a second time, each was interviewed at the National Cancer Institute about general subjects including their marriage, their children, their job, and the cancer. Each then began treatment, which included surgery, radiation, and chemotherapy. Mortality is high among women who get breast cancer a second time, and women in this study began to pass away after about a year—but a small minority survived for much longer. They were the ones whose interview responses showed that they felt "great joy in living" and had chosen optimism.[6]

Optimism, Seligman continued, can protect against depression, heighten your levels of achievement, and boost your physical well-being. In short, "It is a far more pleasant mental state to be in."[7]

So how do we turn away from pessimism and fill our minds and hearts with hope? How do we become "learned optimists"?

Change the Way You Think

The enemy constructs pessimistic strongholds to be like fortresses, each brick a disappointment or betrayal or deeply felt wound. These bricks wall us off from God's purposes for us— they block us from staying in the love walk. The exciting news is that pessimism is a fortress we can tear down and destroy with the tools God has given us. Paul wrote to his young associate in 2 Timothy 1:7, "For God has not given us a spirit of fear, but of power and of love and of a sound mind." He wrote in 2 Corinthians 10:4–5, "For the weapons of our warfare are not carnal but mighty in God for pulling down strongholds, casting down arguments and every high thing that exalts itself against the knowledge of God, bringing every thought into captivity to the obedience of Christ."

In Philippians 4:6–7 (NLT) Paul commanded, "Don't worry about anything; instead, pray about everything. Tell God what you need, and thank him for all he has done. Then you will experience God's peace, which exceeds anything we can understand." He concludes this passage by writing, "Finally, brethren, whatever things are true, whatever things are noble, whatever things are just, whatever things are pure, whatever things are lovely, whatever things are of good report, if there is any virtue and if there is anything praiseworthy—meditate on these things" (v. 8).

God has given us control over our own thoughts. The Bible says, "Let this mind be in you which was also in Christ Jesus" (Phil. 2:5). We are told how to control our thoughts, our beliefs, our explanatory style. It is not the Holy Spirit's job to resist our ungodly thoughts—it's ours. We must take responsibility to banish the ungodly mindsets in which pessimism breeds. When a hopeless thought, an anxious thought, a fearful or depressing thought comes into our minds, we immediately say, "That is not my thought! That is Satan's thought. He is the accuser, the blamer, the ultimate pessimist, and he comes only to steal, kill, and destroy. I am taking that thought captive in obedience to Christ and casting it out of my mind."

Dodie Osteen learned a lot about the power of hope when battling stage IV cancer in her early forties. She tenaciously grabbed on to the hope we have as God's children. "God is for you," she wrote in her book *Healed of Cancer.* "'For all the promises of God in Him are Yes, and in Him Amen, to the glory of God through us.' [2 Corinthians 1:20] If you do not know the Word of God, you need to learn it....Don't condemn yourself if you don't know the Word. Just get in the Bible and seek the Lord, and He will show Himself strong on your behalf."[8]

Dodie also took practical steps to elevate her hope: She placed a picture of herself in her wedding dress by her bed. She also put out a photo of herself riding a horse on vacation. "They bolstered my faith and helped me keep a positive attitude, especially when I was feeling so sick," she writes. "I kept looking at those pictures and saying, 'Thank You, Father, that You will restore health to me and heal me of my wounds. I thank You that I'll feel like I did when I married at 21. I'll feel like I did when I was 25 riding that horse. I thank You that You will restore health to me, Father.'"[9]

Interestingly, cognitive therapy has discovered the effectiveness of the Bible's approach, whether the therapists know it or not! To overcome negative thinking, Seligman suggests the following prescription:

First, learn to identify the automatic negative thoughts that arise when you feel low.

Second, challenge those thoughts by finding evidence that contradicts them.

Third, offer different explanations, or "reattributions," to dispute those automatic thoughts.

Fourth, develop ways to distract yourself from depressing thoughts.

Fifth, learn to recognize and question the underlying assumptions that contribute to your depression.

"Just because a person fears that he is unemployable, unlovable, or inadequate doesn't mean it's true," Seligman says.[10] It's important to take a step back and temporarily suspend belief in your pessimistic thoughts to assess their validity. Then actively challenge and dismantle them [as advised in the Bible]. "Give them an argument," he writes. "Go on the attack. By effectively disputing the beliefs that follow adversity, you can change your customary reaction from dejection and giving up to activity and good cheer."[11]

Secular scientists believe our level of hope, even in the natural, is the result of choice far more than genetic disposition. In an interview with *The New York Times*, Alan Rozanski said that "our way of thinking is habitual, unaware, so the first step is to learn to control ourselves when negative thoughts assail us and commit ourselves to change the way we look at things. We must recognize that our way of thinking is not necessarily the only way of looking at a situation. This thought alone can lower the toxic effect of negativity." Rozanski believes that hope—which he calls "optimism"—can be exercised like a muscle and trained to become stronger as we deliberately replace any irrational negative thoughts with positive ones.[12]

T. L. Osborn illuminated the same principle in his wonderful book *The Message That Works*. "Analyze your thoughts," he said. "If they contradict the facts of redemption, then simply change them. Think redemptive thoughts. Think of what God says. Ponder it. Rejoice in it. Talk it. Communicate it. Believe it. And act on it. Discouragement will dissipate like a toxic fog before the sunshine."[13]

None of this means we should ignore facts in favor of feel-good fantasies and a Pollyanna perspective. God does not counsel us to rely on "the power of positive thinking." No, we are in the business of replacing lies with facts—the facts of our redemption, the fact of our identity in Christ, the facts of the glorious future and powerful present God has prepared for each one of us.

Learned optimism is about being accurate in your thinking, writes Seligman. Negative beliefs that arise after setbacks are often incorrect. Look for evidence that reveals the exaggerations in your negative explanations. Most of the time, reality supports a more positive view: "The most convincing way of disputing a negative belief is to show that it is factually incorrect."[14]

TRUE AND FACTUAL

God's perspective is true and factual, not blind. Pessimism is inaccurate, but habits of negative thinking sometimes take a lot of work to root out. We must be persistent about attacking them, questioning them, holding them up to scrutiny, and then evicting them from our minds and emotions. This is a big part of what the Bible calls crucifying the flesh daily, as it says in Galatians 5:24: "And those who are Christ's have crucified the flesh with its passions and desires."

People can accustom themselves to pessimistic thinking so that it actually becomes desirable to them. They convince themselves that hopelessness protects them from pain, just as alcoholics believe that drinking will make them happier than remaining sober. But we must resist the temptation to abandon hope. Romans 12:2 urges us, "And do not be conformed to this world, but be transformed by the renewing of your mind, that you may prove what is that good and acceptable and perfect will of God." Second Corinthians 5:17 reminds us powerfully, "Therefore, if anyone is in Christ, he is a new creation; old things have passed away; behold, all things have become new."

We must assure ourselves that in Christ, God holds no blame for us, as it reads in Colossians 2:13–15 (NLT):

> You were dead because of your sins and because your sinful nature was not yet cut away. Then God made you alive with Christ, for he forgave all our sins. He canceled the record of the charges against us and took it away by nailing it to the cross. In this way, he disarmed the spiritual rulers and authorities. He shamed them publicly by his victory over them on the cross.

We must grasp and personalize the words of Ephesians 1:7 (AMP), which say, "In Him we have redemption [that is, our deliverance and salvation] through His blood, [which paid the penalty for our sin and resulted in] the forgiveness and complete pardon of our sin, in accordance with the riches of His grace."

We need to forgive ourselves for our failures, real or imagined, and then see ourselves as more than conquerors through Him who loved us, as Romans 8:37 encourages us: "Yet in all these things we are more than conquerors through Him who loved us." We just agree completely with the words of Jesus in John 8:36 (KJV) that "If the Son therefore shall make you free, ye shall be free indeed."

If pessimistic thoughts flood in—such as, "I will never find a good job or meet the right person to marry"—cast them down and say, "No good thing will God withhold to them who walk uprightly." The Word of God has power and authority over all wrong, pessimistic thoughts—but we must exercise it.

We must also eliminate "never" and "always" thinking in any negative sense and boldly put our "always" in the right place. God's Word says, "I can do *all things* through Christ which strengtheneth me" (Phil. 4:13, KJV, emphasis added). With 2 Corinthians 2:14 we confidently affirm, "Now thanks be unto God, which *always* causeth us to triumph in Christ" (KJV, emphasis added). With Philippians 2:5 we say, "I will let this mind be in me which was also in Christ Jesus." Another version puts it this way: "You must have the same attitude that Christ Jesus had" (NLT). With Colossians 1:27 we remind ourselves that the hope of glory resides in us.

The Book of Hebrews gives us an amazing assurance that "we are surrounded by such a huge crowd of witnesses to the life of faith" that we should be bold enough to "strip off every weight [including pessimism] that slows us down, especially the sin that so easily trips us up. And let us run with endurance the race God has set before us. We do this by keeping our eyes on

Jesus, the champion who initiates and perfects our faith" (Heb. 12:1–2, NLT).

As we do this, we can have complete confidence that hope never fails and pessimism can be overcome like any lie of the devil.

IT'S A FACT!

Even secular research confirms that "cognitive therapy works because it changes explanatory style from pessimistic to optimistic, and the change is permanent."[15]

GRATITUDE FUELS HOPE

When hope replaces pessimism, all aspects of our attitudes change, like the sun rising and flooding a landscape with color. One of those changes comes in the area of thankfulness.

Pessimists are almost always ungrateful people. Gratitude and hopefulness go together because gratitude takes us deeper into the love walk where hope and optimism reside in fullness. I like how Robert Emmons and his coauthor, Robin Stern, put it in a paper titled "Gratitude as a Psychotherapeutic Intervention":

A number of rigorous, controlled experimental trials have examined the benefits of gratitude. Gratitude has one of the strongest links to mental health and satisfaction with life of any personality trait—more so than even optimism, hope, or compassion. Grateful people experience higher levels of positive emotions such as joy, enthusiasm, love, happiness, and optimism, and gratitude as a discipline protects us from the destructive impulses of envy, resentment, greed, and bitterness. People who experience gratitude can cope more effectively with everyday stress, show increased resilience in the face of trauma-induced stress, recover more quickly from illness, and enjoy more robust physical health. Taken together, these results indicate that gratitude is incompatible with negative emotions and pathological conditions and that it may even offer protection against psychiatric disorders.[16]

One way researchers scientifically examine the effects of thankfulness is by asking people to keep weekly gratitude journals. Those who did this in one study "exercised more regularly, reported fewer physical symptoms, felt better about their lives as a whole, and were more optimistic about the upcoming week compared with those who recorded hassles or neutral life events."[17] Other benefits included longer sleep and improved sleep quality, and the study participants who kept gratitude journals spent more time exercising.

Even the families and friends of these thankful scribes noted the change in demeanor and reported that "people who practice gratitude seem measurably happier and are more pleasant to be around. Grateful people are rated by others as more helpful, outgoing, optimistic, and trustworthy."[18]

Thanksgiving activates hope. It clears away the mists of self-centeredness and negativity, giving us an elevated and accurate view of the way things are and of the future ahead. So Paul instructed us, "In everything give thanks; for this is the will of God in Christ Jesus for you" (1 Thess. 5:18).

THE HEALING POWER OF JOY

Another close ally of hope is joy. I had a patient die a few weeks ago at the age of 103. This woman walked in divine health, rarely got sick, stayed full of joy and love, and was a powerful prayer warrior. I talked with her daughter shortly after she went to be with the Lord, and the daughter said that in the days before her death, her mom had been in the hospital wearing her little gown when the therapist came to walk her to the therapy room. By this time she was wearing adult diapers and her body was giving out—but still she started dancing a jig and singing right there in the hallway. The nurses in attendance could not believe it. The joy of the Lord was manifesting right in front of them. That was someone living fully in God's love walk. A few days later she went to sleep and went home to be with the Lord.

Joy is an inside job. We've probably all known self-described Christians who scramble around trying to find joy in hobbies, jobs, relationships, career advancement, money, risk-taking adventures, gambling, leisure activities, and more. They go home after work and spend hours playing video games or cycle endlessly from football season to basketball season to baseball season.

These pursuits can provide a diversion or an immediate rush of excitement, but the effect is ephemeral—it does not last. It builds no durable strength, and the "joy" fizzles away rapidly. No new car, new house, beautiful or handsome spouse, money, prestige, power, sex, fun, or success can fill your joy tank for long if you don't have joy in your heart already. But when we remain in the love walk, we unleash joy unspeakable and full of glory, as the apostle Peter wrote in 1 Peter 1:8 (KJV).

One of the most joy-filled, down-to-earth people I know is Andrew Wommack, founder of Charis Bible College near Colorado Springs, Colorado. Andrew is an extraordinary man and the first to say he comes across like some country boy from *The Andy Griffith Show*. A Texan by birth, he pastored three very small churches and also started a radio ministry, but when he was in his fifties the Lord corrected him strongly through Psalm 78:41 and said he was limiting God with small thinking. Andrew repented and opened his mind and heart to the greater things God wanted to do through him, and today he has Charis Bible College campuses all over the world, employs more than a thousand people, and has a billion dollars in projects going.

Over the years, Andrew has prayed for and seen multiple people raised from the dead, including one of his sons, who was in the morgue with a toe tag and had been dead for five hours.[19] He also knows the Bible like nobody I know.

Best of all, Andrew is full of joy. He doesn't put on airs of any type. If you saw him walking around the campus of the college he leads, you might think he was the janitor because he doesn't exude pride or self-importance. Rather, his life is about serving other people. He embodies the love and joy of God like no other friend I have, and being with him is so refreshing. To me, it's like spending time with the Lord as a friend. When I meet someone who needs to spend time in the presence of God, I send them to Andrew's ministry campus in Woodland Park, Colorado.

IT'S A FACT!

The key to joy in life is receiving the love of God and then giving that love to others. Christians should be the most joyful people on earth. Since the love of God has been shed abroad in your heart by the Holy Spirit, and not in your head or your feelings, that love is the same love God loves you with—an unselfish love with fullness of joy.

Andrew often says, "I'm not the sharpest tool in the tool chest. I would not have been God's first choice. I'm just a simple man and don't even have a college education. But I believe God and know His Word." Recently a Muslim woman in England experienced an angelic visitation, and the angel told her, "If you want to see God, go to this address." She went to that address, and it was Charis Bible College's campus in London! The joy and love there are like beacons in a dark world, and Andrew is a great example of how the most joyful life is the unselfish life.

In His great message on love, Jesus connected love to joy, saying in John 15:11–12, "These things I have spoken to you, that My joy may remain in you, and that your joy may be full. This is My commandment, that you love one another as I have loved you." He made a direct connection between the two attributes. Psalm 16:11 tells us that in God's presence is fullness of joy. Nehemiah 8:10 says the joy of the Lord is our strength.

An Extra Dose of Joy

My grandson Braden has exhibited unusual levels of joy since he was a baby, so much so that Mary and I gave him the nickname "Joy Boy." Even as a toddler Braden would go up to a new kid and hug him or her. This happened everywhere we went. To this day he loves to laugh. He comes and works out with me, and we spend much of the time laughing. Our other grandchildren are joyful too, but Braden seems to have an extra dose of it.

In my practice I spend some days feeling like I am pumping people up with joy only to watch their attitudes go flat again like the tires on an old bicycle. Hope and joy sustain each other; you really can't have one without the other. This is why Paul could say in Philippians 4:11 that he had learned how to be happy at all times. He never gave in to hopelessness or a pessimistic viewpoint. I was reading 2 Corinthians 11 recently, where Paul was recounting the trials he went through and yet his joy was irrepressible. He didn't personalize, universalize, or catastrophize his tribulations. He was not overwhelmed by stress or seeing a therapist for years for a bad case of PTSD. "Rejoice in the Lord always," he wrote. "Again I will say, rejoice!" (Phil. 4:4). This was Paul's teaching and his personal practice. Joy was his strength, along with unshakable hope.

Likewise, David declared in Psalm 34:1, "I will bless the LORD at all times; His praise shall continually be in my mouth." Many Christians claim to have joy, but most have not notified their faces yet! John Hagee said many Christians look like they have been baptized in pickle juice. But when we follow Jesus' command to love one another, a primary result will be fullness of joy. When we wear a smile and bubble up with joy, the world will want to know what we have and what they are missing. Love your neighbors as yourself. For your joy to be full, simply walk in love toward everyone.

Look a little closer at the connection Jesus made between the two in John 15:9–13 (emphasis added):

> As the Father loved Me, I also have loved you; abide in My love. If you keep My commandments, you will abide in My love, just as I have kept My Father's commandments and abide in His love. *These things I have spoken to you, that My joy may remain in you, and that your joy may be full.* This is My commandment, that you love one another as I have loved you. Greater love has no one than this, than to lay down one's life for his friends.

But what things had Jesus spoken of so that His joy would remain in them and their joy would be full? Simply look at the preceding verse, John 15:10 (NLT): "When you obey my commandments, you remain in my love, just as I obey my Father's commandments and remain in his love." Remember Galatians 5:14 (NLT), "For the whole law can be summed up in this one commandment: 'Love your neighbor as yourself.'"

If we don't have joy, are we really walking in God's love? Jesus had joy even as His soul was in distress. He taught His friends about love and joy just a few hours before the Romans crucified Him on a cross. Do you have joy in your distress? We must. This is the higher reality of God's love. If we are not overcoming every pessimistic thought that comes at us with love, hope, and the joy of God, we are living beneath our birthright as sons and daughters of the King—and we are not choosing the best for our own health.

As a doctor, I like the word *strength*. My patients talk often about wanting to maintain strength to perform physical exercise, pick up their children and grandchildren, build things and engage in hobbies, or even just get out of bed in the morning and take a shower on their own.

Strength has so many meanings and manifestations, and joy fuels them all. Joy gives us strength to overcome adversity and the ability to bear up under persecution or difficult circumstances. It gives us the fortitude to make right decisions about our diet and medical choices. Joy is power, and Paul wrote about having power, love, and a sound mind (2 Tim. 1:7). This is another way of saying that joy and love help us make sound decisions that promote a healthy lifestyle, a healthy body, healthy emotions, and so on. All of this flows from love.

If our joy is not full, we may not be loving others selflessly enough. Jesus said that even godless people love each other, but it is not selfless love. Rather, "Greater love has no one than this, than to lay down one's life for his friends" (John 15:13). Love is most powerful when it is selfless, and this God kind of love leads to "fullness of joy."

I have known many great leaders, but only a few walked in a joy that radiates. One who did so was Kenneth Hagin; he always looked as if he had just heard a great joke or story. To me, his face reflected the joy of heaven. T. L. Osborn was the other who glowed with the joy of the Lord. It emanated from his eyes and permeated his speech. That level of joy, love, and hope was something I had never seen before. "Lord, this is how we're all supposed to be," I said to myself when I met him. All of us are made to have joy sparkling in our eyes, bounces in our steps, songs in our mouths, and hearts brimming with hopeful anticipation of God's good future.

DEVELOP HEALTHY, HOPE-FILLED AMBITIONS

Hope always has an element of desire to it. T. L. Osborn wrote about this:

> Buddha taught that human persons could achieve a level of mental control where all desires in life would be neutralized and that the very root of desire would die....It is like trying to cure a headache by getting rid of the head. We are created with the emotional capacity to admire what is beautiful, good and productive. God wants those healthy emotions in you freed so you can soar to new levels and bless your world on a scale which religious prejudice would forbid you to even dream about.[20]

He then wrote with great insight that "since the day God created Adam and Eve in an environment of abundance, happiness, health and fulfillment, He has never changed His mind about people. You have the miraculous capacity that no other creature has—to think and plan, to ponder and imagine, to believe and achieve, to acquire what you desire."[21]

Pessimism squelches desire, because desire can disappoint—but we are not imprisoned in the delusion of pessimism. We break free of it with boundless hope.

Osborn put it this way:

> God wants you to realize that within you is the possibility to shed the cloak of failure, to escape the negative syndrome of discouragement, to break with the demoralizing dogmas of defeat, to get out of the boredom of conformity and to go for life at its best. Aspire to more than the average person settles for. A common characteristic of all winners is, they deeply aspire to win. The force of eager aspiration in you has a miraculous way of releasing powerful energy, creativity and an almost supernatural pull toward what you yearn for. One of the most vital facts you will discover is that God wants you to have good things—the best in life, but He must wait until you aspire to have them, and go for them before He can give them to you.[22]

Hopeful desire is your destiny. It helps move us forward in the love walk with confidence and expectation. The Bible commands that we strip off everything that hinders our forward progress, including pessimism. We do so in an attitude of faith—the other primary partner of love, which we will talk about in the next chapter.

PRAYER AND DECLARATIONS

Father, I reject pessimism entirely and all its corrosive, dampening effects on my soul, my ambitions, and my life. I choose to believe the best about my future, about Your intentions for me, and about what I can achieve. Help me to make the decision throughout each day to choose to believe in hope; to cast down every thought that exalts itself against the knowledge of You; and to uproot bad habits of thought and behavior that undermine my progress in the love walk. I will no longer seek to protect myself with the false shield of pessimism and low expectations. Rather, I will rejoice in hopeful expectation, letting the joy of the Lord be my strength as I seek to do everything from an attitude of selfless love. Amen.

In honor of this joy-filled man, let me share one of T. L. Osborn's lists of declarations, which I have modified to serve the format of this book. Start by saying out loud, "From today, no person or demon or religion or system is going to restrict and restrain me, condemn and confuse me, judge and abuse me, or manipulate and maneuver me."

Now declare:

I deserve God's best because He created it for me.

I deserve good news because He sends it to me.

I deserve total happiness because He fashioned me.

I deserve exhilarating health because He is in me.

I deserve unlimited prosperity because His goodness is all around me.

I deserve genuine love because He forgave me.

I deserve a positive uplift because He inspires me.

I am made for life and not for death.

I am made for health and not for disease.

I am made for success and not for failure.

I am made for faith and not for confusion.

I am made for love and not for fear.

I am discovering that God wants my life to represent all of the good that He is and that He has created.

I have done what Jesus said to do:
I have sought first the kingdom of God.
I have discovered that God and I are coworkers in His powerful love-plan.
I have accepted His promise that all of these good things shall be added to me (Matt. 6:33).
I have learned to see myself like God sees me.
I have discovered the wonder of His grace.

I have learned to affirm:
I am part of God's plan.
I am an instrument in His kingdom. I am a member of His family.
I am the proof of God's love. I am the evidence of His life. I am the form of His body.
I am the temple of His Spirit.
I am the expression of God's faith. I am the fruit of His life.

I am the action of His plan.
God made me.
God believes in me.
God loves me.
God paid for me.
God never gave up on me. God gave His Son for me.
God redeemed me.
God values me.
I am breathing fresh air. I am hearing new music. A new song is born in me.[23]

I was created for love, and love exists for me.

My desire for love is God's desire in me for His love to flow through me to lift and to bless everyone, proving He lives in me.

From today, God's new, nonjudgmental love will begin to rule in my life and to pour out to others through me.[24]

CHAPTER 11

SPEAKING LIFE

KENNETH COPELAND BECAME my patient in the late 1990s, and I will never forget the first time he visited my office for a consultation. I had met Kenneth before and been edified by his ministry for years. Now I was looking forward to serving him in my professional capacity as a doctor. In advance of our appointment I ordered bloodwork and the usual tests that help indicate if anything unhealthy is going on in one's body. On the day of our appointment I came into the room and greeted Kenneth. After we chatted a little bit, I began to talk about his test results.

When I was done with some preliminary observations, he said something that, though spoken very gently, stunned me.

"Dr. Colbert," he said, "would you mind rephrasing that statement and put faith in it?"

Flustered and feeling a bit rebuked, I stammered, "Sure, I'm sorry."

"No, you're not sorry," he said. "'Sorry' means you're a good-for-nothing person. You are not a good-for-nothing person. You can apologize, but don't say you are sorry."

"I'm—" I started to say reflexively, then completed the sentence, "I apologize."

All my professional pride went right out the door, and standing there in my white lab coat I felt two inches tall. Kenneth smiled, and I knew he meant no harm or disrespect.

"Don," he told me, "every word that comes out of your mouth needs to be a faith-filled word. There can be no negativity."

I nodded and said, "Yes, you're right." I considered myself a faith-filled person, but this was next-level faith.

Recentering myself and looking at my notes, I began to try to speak about the test data using only words of faith, but at times I found myself falling back into descriptions I typically used with other patients. For example, at one point I said, "One of your lab values is a little out of range."

"What does that mean?" Kenneth asked.

"It means that your level of inflammation is mildly elevated, which could increase your risk of heart disease or stroke," I answered.

"Please rephrase that for me with faith," he said.

I paused to think for a moment, then restated it: "This lab value is just a little out of range. It should come down with the food and supplement changes I suggest, and I will recheck it in six months."

"That's better," he said.

Kenneth became my patient and friend from that day forward, but I had to learn to watch every word that came out of my mouth whenever he visited my office. It was anything but easy. My pride often stung. My carnal mind screamed to justify itself. I frequently felt like I was on the witness stand, with each of my words being examined under a faith microscope. One time he told me kindly but firmly, "Don, you are unknowingly cursing me and cursing your own self when you speak those words. Quit cursing yourself and quit cursing me."

Imagine one of God's generals rebuking you like that! Numerous times in my office with Kenneth I had to back up, say something differently, and identify what I had said that was not of faith. Some appointments took two hours so I could fix my speech. Seldom had I undergone a more rigorous training to speak life rather than death. But while having Kenneth as a patient helped to crucify my flesh, I submitted to it and listened to him—and I'm so glad I did. It might seem like he was hard on me, but his training did me a world of good and my other patients a lot of good.

Over time I caught on to his way of speaking and, more importantly, his way of thinking and living by faith. I learned how to watch every word that comes out of my mouth and to phrase things so they contain no doubt and no unbelief. Up till then I had not realized that my way of explaining medical results and possibilities was sabotaging my faith, hope, and love, and that of my patients.

God—and Kenneth Copeland—loved me enough to help me go higher. As a result of that godly correction, I walk in greater expectancy and faith than ever before.

By the way, Mary loved my "training" under Kenneth Copeland. "You are being so molded by this!" she gushed. Easy for her to say!

ACTUALIZING OUR EXPECTATIONS

Faith is integral to the love walk and living a life that is pleasing to God. Without faith it is impossible to please God, Hebrews 11:6 tells us. "The just shall live by faith," Paul wrote (Rom. 1:17), and in another place he said, "For we walk by faith, not by sight" (2 Cor. 5:7). Our salvation comes through faith, as it says, "For by grace you have been saved through faith" (Eph. 2:8). Paul also exhorted us to "fight the good fight of faith, lay hold on eternal life, to which you were also called and have confessed the good confession in the presence of many witnesses" (1 Tim. 6:12). "And this," the apostle John agrees, "is the victory that has overcome the world—our faith" (1 John 5:4).

Clearly there is no such thing as faithless Christianity. Each believer must be "building yourselves up on your most holy faith, praying in the Holy Spirit" (Jude 20). Romans 12:3 promises that God has given to every person a measure of faith—and it is entirely up to us how we use it.

Faith, hope, and love are like three strands of an eternal cord. They interconnect and work together in our lives. Hebrews 11:1 tells us, "Now faith is the substance of things hoped for, the evidence of things not seen." This tells us that faith manifests the things we hope for. It actualizes our godly expectations, and in truth there is no faith without hope. Neither is there faith without love, as Galatians 5:6 (NIV) says, "The only thing that counts is faith expressing itself through love."

We looked earlier at what love and hope are, but what is faith? Faith is not a feeling but an act of the will to say, "God has a good outcome in mind and the power to fulfill it." Faith is based on facts, not wishes and dreams. Faith produces in the natural the things we hope for. Believe it or not, this principle is universal and works even for the ungodly. I recently watched a documentary about cryptocurrency in which a thieving scoundrel conned people out of millions of dollars with a scheme. What caught my attention was that this man always confessed he would be rich. He saw himself as rich, he expected to get rich, and it happened. He used faith principles, and they worked for him.

But to use faith in its proper way, we must pair it with love.

Jesus said that if we love Him we will obey His commandments (John 4:15), so obedience is an act of faith motivated by love. Paul told us to "Fight the good fight of faith, [and] lay hold on eternal life, to which you were also called and have confessed the good confession in the presence of many witnesses" (1 Tim. 6:12). T. L. Osborn put it this way: "Faith also involves speaking a good confession. This is our only fight—the faith-fight. It means that we fight to believe what God says and that we resist voices, imaginations, messages, circumstances, concepts, false prophecies, and any other information, factual or illusory, that contradicts the Word. John says, 'This is the victory that overcomes the world, even our faith' (1 John 5:4). Faith in what? Faith in what God's Word says—faith in the victory of Christ over all the works of the devil (1 John 3:8)."[1]

If you think about it, everybody has faith in something, meaning they expect some type of outcome. Some put faith in money, others in relationships or societal influence. Pessimists put faith in bad outcomes, and that faith is powerful and helps bring about negative results. The enemy's goal is to convince us to put our faith anywhere but in God and His Word. "Satan's oppressing spirits will relentlessly tempt and pressure Christians, deceiving them, tricking them, diverting them by delusions and chicanery," Osborn wrote. "He will oppress their bodies with pain and disease and their minds with negative and doubtful thoughts that contradict God's Word. The believer's recourse is to resist the devil (with the facts of the Word of God) and he will flee from you" (James 4:7).[2]

Satan has no control over our faith. He cannot dictate what we believe or expect. He must convince people to misplace their own faith. His only power is in persuasion, and he "can only devour those who believe his lies because they do not know the victory that Christ accomplished on their behalf," Osborn concluded. "They are uninformed so they naively accept Satan's lies as fact."[3]

Where we aim our faith will determine every outcome we experience in life.

Prophesy the Future

Faith is not simply believing in our heads. God has ordained that faith must be spoken with our mouths. God demonstrated this by creating the world through the speaking of words, and likewise all the words we speak have creative power because we are created in His image. In fact, words are the most powerful tool on earth. The Bible tells us words have the power to build up and bless and to tear down and destroy. Jesus said in Matthew 12:32 that "anyone who speaks a word against the Son of Man, it will be forgiven him; but whoever speaks against the Holy Spirit, it will not be forgiven him, either in this age or in the age to come." Our words are so powerful they can rob us of heaven!

In Mark 11:22–24 Jesus taught us that faith is voice-activated, not simply a matter of belief. He said:

> Have faith in God. For assuredly, I say to you, whoever says to this mountain, "Be removed and be cast into the sea," and does not doubt in his heart, but believes that those things he says will be done, he will have whatever he says. Therefore I say to you, whatever things you ask when you pray, believe that you receive them, and you will have them.

Notice how many times Jesus used the word *say* in that brief passage. Our faith must be spoken. The great faith preacher and author Charles Capps was a patient of mine toward the end of his life. He had written a great book called *The Tongue: A Creative Force*. I got to see this man of God walk those principles out, which I believe extended his life. He spoke words of faith right up to the end of his long and productive life. It was a blessing to be around him because even though he had medical issues, he was still speaking the Word by faith. He lived Paul's admonition in Ephesians 4:29 (KJV), "Let no corrupt communication proceed out of your mouth." Corrupt words include not just mean words or off-color jokes but anything that does not agree with God's Word.

Many of us install alarm systems in our homes or cars to keep intruders or thieves out, but how many of us put the same amount of effort to place a guard on our mouths so that no corrupt communication proceeds from them? Psalm 141:3 says wisely, "Set a guard, O LORD, over my mouth; keep watch over the door of my lips." A true and effective Christian will not curse himself with his tongue but will love himself by his words and speak life to his body, mind, and emotions.

Have you ever wondered why the birth of Jesus was spoken beforehand by the prophets? It is because of this principle of speaking things into existence. The prophets had to speak the coming of Jesus so that Jesus could come! This very same principle operates in our lives today. We must speak realities before they manifest. "If you confess with your mouth the Lord Jesus and believe in your heart that God has raised Him from the dead, you will be saved," Paul wrote to the Romans, "for with the heart one believes unto righteousness, and with the mouth confession is made unto salvation" (Rom. 10:9–10).

Our mouths always speak forth what will happen in our lives. "But who do you say that I am?" Jesus asked His disciples (Matt.

16:15). He made them confess who He was before they became His evangelists to the world to declare that very truth. In 1 Timothy 6, Paul used some form of the word "confess" three times when writing to Timothy:

> Fight the good fight of faith, lay hold on eternal life, to which you were also called and have *confessed* the good *confession* in the presence of many witnesses. I urge you in the sight of God who gives life to all things, and before Christ Jesus who witnessed the good *confession* before Pontius Pilate.
>
> —1 TIMOTHY 6:12–13, EMPHASIS ADDED

We fight the good fight of faith by confessing with our mouths what God's Word says about any situation and agreeing with His words and believing them in our hearts. Confession is central to the exercise of Christian faith. Why? Because our words prophesy our future. Even Jesus verbalized His faith in His darkest moment: "And when Jesus had cried out with a loud voice, He said, 'Father, "into Your hands I commit My spirit"'" (Luke 23:46).

What an act of faith to declare that while dying! Confession releases the promises of God. Faith-filled, hope-filled, and love-filled words must flow from our tongues like fresh water at all times. That is why Paul continually told the young churches to encourage one another, to sing songs, hymns, and spiritual songs to each other, to speak only that which builds up. Peter commanded, "If anyone speaks, let him speak as the oracles of God" (1 Pet. 4:11). Hebrews 3:1 tells us to "consider the Apostle and High Priest of our confession, Christ Jesus." Our job is to confess Him—not ourselves or our own selfish thoughts.

Oral Roberts, who was also a patient of mine, told me

something priceless. He said, "When I talk to someone, I always listen to how many times he says, 'I,' 'me,' or 'my.' When I hear him saying that a lot, I know that person is selfish and I have to have caution with him." Roberts also employed another test: He waited to see how long it took for the name of Jesus to come out of a person's mouth, then listened to how often that person said the name of Jesus in conversation. "The more they do, the more I know that person can be trusted," Roberts told me.

The Eternal Weight of Words

The Christian life is largely a battle for our words, which express faith in one thing or another. Satan is always trying to get us to speak words that curse us and open doors for his rule. He did this with Adam and Eve in the beginning. If they had kept their faith in God rather than in the words of the serpent, life on this planet would be radically different. Instead, Adam and Eve shifted their faith away from life and into the realm of death.

Likewise, the millions of Israelites under Moses complained and lost faith on the day they were supposed to enter the Promised Land. If they had simply agreed with the good report of Joshua and Caleb, the entire Old Testament and salvation history would be different, but the Israelites agreed with the bad report of the ten doubtful spies. "So all the congregation lifted up their voices and cried, and the people wept that night" (Num. 14:1). They said, "If only we had died in this wilderness!" (v. 2). And guess what? They did! God gave them what they had spoken, telling Moses, "Say to them, 'As I live,' says the LORD, 'just as you have spoken in My hearing, so I will do to you: The carcasses of you who have complained against Me shall fall in this wilderness'" (vv. 28–29).

Far too many Christians these days do the same thing, prophesying calamity into their lives, opening doors wide to the voice of the enemy, speaking death words instead of God's life words. They literally give the enemy of their souls access and control over their future by the power of their misplaced faith. Too many Christians I see in my practice default to speaking their fears, not their God-intended futures. They run on at the mouth like the world does and go through life putting their faith in negative outcomes, confessing unwanted futures, and losing battles.

Jesus warned against speaking "idle words," meaning unproductive words: "But I say to you that for every idle word men may speak, they will give account of it in the day of judgment. For by your words you will be justified, and by your words you will be condemned" (Matt. 12:36–37). The Amplified version calls them "careless or useless" words. Idle words are empty and powerless. They use energy for no good purpose, distract us from what God says or intends in a given situation, and lead us and others to make mistakes. Proverbs tells us that "in the multitude of words sin is not lacking, but he who restrains his lips is wise" (10:19).

Zechariah, the father of John the Baptist, did not restrain his lips but spoke faithless words that caused the angel Gabriel to strike him mute until he was willing once again to speak God's outcome by faith. (See Luke 1.) Zechariah questioned if a son could really be born to him and his wife, seeing as they were old. Perhaps his faithless words could have cursed God's purposes and caused them to be stillborn. In any case, the response was quick and severe: Gabriel shut Zechariah's mouth! If he hadn't, maybe John the Baptist would not have been born as promised.

(See Luke 1:18–20.) Such is the power we exercise in our words of agreement and disagreement.

Unfortunately most Christians I interact with treat words as cheap or nonbinding, things to be thrown around without consequence. Psalm 12:2–4 describes them this way:

> They speak idly everyone with his neighbor; with flattering lips and a double heart they speak. May the LORD cut off all flattering lips, and the tongue that speaks proud things, who have said, "With our tongue we will prevail; our lips are our own; who is lord over us?"

That should convict some of us! When we claim that our words belong to us and can be spoken without any negative results, we deceive ourselves. If the Lord is not the Lord over our tongues, then He is not Lord over us. It is far better to be quiet than to speak idle words. We must consider what we say before we say it. If it does not minister grace to the hearer (Eph. 4:29), we should get good at biting our tongues because those words can become tools of Satan. On the other hand, words that agree with God become tools of angels to bring blessings into our lives.

IT'S A FACT!

"The words you say will either acquit you or condemn you," Jesus said (Matt. 12:37, NLT). Your words carry more weight than you realize.

Some people have been taught to always express their feelings, but in giving their tongues free rein they spend their days tearing down other people and aborting God's plans. Do yourself a favor: avoid speaking your feelings. Feelings so often lie.

Instead, speak the truth Jesus said in John 6:63: "The words that I speak to you are spirit, and they are life." Speak spirit words that bring life. Speak words of faith, hope, and love. Paul wrote:

> Finally, brethren, whatever things are true, whatever things are noble, whatever things are just, whatever things are pure, whatever things are lovely, whatever things are of good report, if there is any virtue and if there is anything praiseworthy—meditate on these things.
>
> —PHILIPPIANS 4:8

We must meditate on good things because our meditations eventually come out of our mouths, as David wrote:

> Let the words of my mouth and the meditation of my heart be acceptable in Your sight, O LORD, my strength and my Redeemer.
>
> —PSALM 19:14

> Death and life are in the power of the tongue, and those who love it will eat its fruit.
>
> —PROVERBS 18:21

WORDS LIKE SWORDS

When I was a boy, I used to watch the old show *The Honeymooners* starring Jackie Gleason when I visited my grandmother and grandfather. Back then, the actors' bickering and banter seemed funny to me, but nowadays it causes a knot in my stomach. It is full of strife, and that show and many others depict people freely belittling one another and cutting people down. It feels like piercings to my soul, as the Word says: "There is one who speaks like the piercings of a sword, but the tongue of the wise promotes health" (Prov. 12:18).

A story is told of a woman whose words were such "piercings." She would not reform her tongue, and so her pastor took her to the top of a local building and told her to open a pillow full of feathers. She did so, and the feathers flew everywhere. Then he instructed her to gather all the feathers—an impossibility since there were so many and they were scattered about. The feathers, he said, represented the words she spoke. Once released, they could not be taken back. That is a powerful picture for us as well.[4]

Other Christians don't pierce with their words but rather go through life speaking mixed messages to themselves and others. They offer lip service to God's promises, quoting Bible verses and such. But they mingle it with worldly wisdom, little aphorisms like "God helps those who help themselves," which is not found in the Bible, and other phrases. Their goal is to be "balanced," "cautious," and "realistic," but in the attempt they offset the promises of God by hedging their language.

They say things such as, "You never know how things will turn out. Sometimes we don't get what we want. It is better to hope for the best and expect the worst." Instead of using the power of words for good, for themselves and others, they equivocate their way through life. They are the picture of what the apostle James, brother of Jesus, called double-minded people, those who entertain opposing thoughts and as a result never get anywhere. He described them as people tossed about like waves on the sea, going back and forth with energy but never arriving anywhere. This is what happens when we "balance" our faith with realism. Having a "balanced" perspective is a sophisticated way of saying we combine faith with doubt. James says such people can expect to receive nothing from the Lord.

Instead, we must speak faith boldly! In His earthly ministry Jesus often made people speak their desire to be healed. Only then did He heal them, saying things like, "According to your faith let it be to you" (Matt. 9:29). We must not waffle between words of faith and "realistic" words of lowered expectations. Hebrews 10:23 says our job is to "hold fast the confession of our hope without wavering."

The sobering fact is that if you do everything else right but get your words wrong, you will not get very far in life. By watching our words, we activate our faith. Here's a challenge for you: Listen to yourself for a day and see how many times you curse yourself with your tongue. Pay attention to how much of what you say is trivial, faith-eroding talk or some attempt to "balance" your perspective with realism. An untamed tongue can stymie everything else we do, even if we are living right in so many other ways.

We will look more at the life-changing power of faith in the next chapter.

PRAYER AND DECLARATIONS

Father, forgive me for the idle words I have spoken. I lay them at Your feet and commit now to speaking only words of faith, hope, and love. Help me to prophesy Your future for myself and others; to speak life and not death; to utter words that build up and not words that are like the piercings of a sword. Thank You that You created me with the ability to literally speak life, as You do. Death and life are in the power of the tongue, and I choose to speak life over myself and everyone I meet. Amen.

I will use the power of my tongue to speak life, to edify, to encourage, to offer hope, to strengthen faith, and to express love.

I renounce low expectations and doubt, which weaken my words. I speak the truth boldly without "balancing" it with doubt.

In accordance with Psalm 34:13, I keep my lips from speaking evil.

I speak life over my family, my work, my ministry endeavors, my imagination, my hobbies, my meditations, and every other aspect of my life.

CHAPTER 12

FAITH AND HEALING ARE VOICE-ACTIVATED

EALING AND SALVATION through Jesus Christ happen the same way: through the confession of faith. God has made our mouths the mechanism by which health and life are gained or lost. So Proverbs 18:21 says, "Death and life are in the power of the tongue, and those who love it will eat its fruit." Jesus warned in Matthew 12:37, "For by your words you will be justified, and by your words you will be condemned." Proverbs 21:23 tells us, "Whoever guards his mouth and tongue keeps his soul from troubles."

I shared earlier about how Dodie Osteen was given a death sentence by a doctor when she was still in her forties. It started when she and John were invited to Oral Roberts University for the opening of the City of Faith and Dodie began having chills and fever, then jaundice. A Houston doctor ran some tests on her and met John in the hallway with devastating news: "Your wife has only a few weeks to live."

Dodie told me about the struggle that ensued, and she wrote in her book, "I had never been a fearful person. But when cancer tried to attach itself to my body, I had to fight fear. Now you may think that seems strange, coming from a pastor's wife, and from a Holy Spirit-filled Christian. I don't try to justify it or reason it out. I'm just telling you how it was with me so it might help you. I'm a human being, and the same things come against me that come against anybody else. So I had to fight fear. And I did it with verses like 2 Timothy 1:7. I would say, 'Father, You haven't given me the spirit of fear, but of power and of love and of a sound mind. This fear is not of You, God. It's of the devil. So I'm commanding it to leave now, in Jesus' Name.'"[1]

The Osteen family had many faith-filled friends such as Oral Roberts, Kenneth Hagin, Kenneth Copeland, T. L. Osborn, and others. John asked them to come pray for Dodie's healing, and they did, but one night in the wee hours God spoke to Dodie and said, "It is not the faith of any of these men but your own that you must go on now." She redoubled her efforts to fight the fight of faith with her own words and confession.

She wrote, "I set a date, September 6, as the day I believed I would be free of the torment of fear. I said, 'From this day, I shall have no more fear. It's gone, in Jesus' Name.' If fear is coming against you, rebuke it. Say, 'On this day, the day I am reading these words, I'm getting rid of fear. Fear, release me in Jesus' Name. You have no right to torment a child of God. I am full of his peace and love. Now, I cast all my care upon You, Father, because I know You care for me. And I thank You that I am free from fear. Fear may come, but faith overrules it.'"[2]

I am inspired just reading those powerful words. Of course she paired them with actions and was very practical about it. Upon arriving home from the hospital, she did not go to bed or ask others to wait on her. "I felt that if I did, it would demonstrate unbelief and undermine my faith," she wrote. "I went to bed only at night during normal sleeping hours. I wouldn't even take a nap."[3]

One time in those difficult days of fighting the fight of faith for her health, Dodie wanted a small piece of furniture in a room moved to another spot. It would have been no problem for her to do when she was healthy, but it was not easy in her physical condition at the time. But when she asked her children for help, one of them said, "Mother, you are healed. You can do it." The kids would not help their mother! Rather, they were determined to help her in another way—to stand on faith for her healing.

Dodie was irritated at first by their unwillingness, but it caused her to move the furniture herself. Sure, it felt hard, but it made her exercise her faith. "I thank God [our children] have been grounded in the Word of God," she reflected afterward. "Don't sit around and feel sorry for yourself when you are fighting the battle for your healing. Pity never wins! I overcame my pity parties by speaking to my body and commanding it to come in line with the Word of God. And it did!"[4]

BE READY TO FIGHT

The fight of faith is just that—a fight—and we face setbacks on the way to victory.

"I wavered many times," Dodie wrote. "Of course, it was in my mind, my thoughts, not in my heart! Those accusations that come against you in your mind are from the evil one. The devil is the one who is the accuser of the brethren (see Revelation 12:10). When he tells you anything, believe just the opposite, and you'll have the truth. I learned not to condemn myself any more. I would say, 'I thank You, Father, that I am holding fast to my confession without wavering. I don't waver in my spirit man because I know Your Word works.'"[5]

As a registered nurse, she understood very well how her body was supposed to function, and she understood that it was not functioning properly—a potentially frightening circumstance. "Certain things the doctors had said now brought fear to my heart," she wrote. "Those were the thoughts I had to fight against most, and I still have to resist them sometimes. Satan would torment me with the doctor's words, 'You have only a few weeks to live...few weeks to live...few weeks to live.' He would use pain and then say, 'You're going to die. Have your family bury you in that pretty pink dress. You look good in it.'... The devil bombarded my mind with every kind of fear imaginable, especially when everybody was asleep and I lay awake. Symptoms came against my body, mostly demonic and tormenting thoughts, just to try my faith."[6]

She spoke the Word of God over her body every day, passages like Psalm 91:14–16, which says:

> Because he has set his love upon Me, therefore I will deliver him; I will set him on high, because he has known My name. He shall call upon Me, and I will answer him; I will be with him in trouble; I will deliver him and honor him. With long life I will satisfy him, and show him My salvation.

And Psalm 118:17, which reads:

> I shall not die, but live, and declare the works of the LORD.

One verse that became life to her was Philippians 2:13, which says, "for it is God who works in you both to will and to do for His good pleasure." "This verse has sustained me in many dark hours," she wrote. "When I'm driving my car or out for a walk, it just rolls out, over and over. I say, 'God, you said that You are working in me. You are working in my body both to will and to do for Your good pleasure. Father, You are working in my mind, renewing it. My health is your good pleasure.'...This will help you, too. If you feel like you are wavering, remember this: you can have doubt in your head but still have faith in your heart.... If you are believing God for something, watch what comes out of your mouth. Keep on confessing the Word of God, and God will honor His Word."[7]

Dodie discovered that it is useless to fight negative thoughts and lies only with thoughts. It does not even help to simply replace a negative thought with a positive thought. No—faith is voice-activated, as we have seen. When we find ourselves in a struggle for our lives, or even in everyday situations, we must replace negative thoughts with godly thoughts and then speak them out of our mouths. Do you feel sick? "Let the weak say, 'I am strong'" (Joel 3:10). Speak Matthew 8:17, which says, "He Himself took our infirmities and bore our sicknesses."

You know the outcome: Dodie has lived another forty-three years and is still going at the printing of this book. And she was given only two months to live with stage IV metastatic liver cancer!

A patient came into my office whom I had seen six months earlier. In the interim she had come down with shingles and broken out in horrible blisters on her abdomen. She was in terrible pain, and her local hospital had given her several antiviral medicines. She went home and suddenly remembered, "Wait, I have a covenant with God!" She called to mind the many scriptures that promise healing, and she got mad at the devil. She started rebuking the enemy and confessing healing scriptures, and her body began healing within hours. The pain went away, and she did not have to take the antiviral medications doctors had prescribed for her.

I like how Osborn put it: "Faith means you link yourself with God, even when you cannot see Him or feel Him. Faith means you believe His promises, and you pray, and receive the answer in a way that no one can explain."[8]

WHEN OUR OWN WORDS CONDEMN US

The enemy tries to stifle our faith by tricking us into self-con-demnation. His goal is to rob our words of power and under-mine our success in Christ. When we doubt God's words, we waver. We lose confidence, and our faith becomes ineffective. As John wrote,

> For if our heart condemns us, God is greater than our heart, and knows all things. Beloved, if our heart does not condemn us, we have confidence toward God. And what-ever we ask we receive from Him.
>
> —1 JOHN 3:20–22

Anything that undermines our confidence disempowers our words. This includes not believing our own words, because many Christians joke and tell "white lies." For example, if we tell someone we will meet them at 7 p.m. for dinner knowing we can't arrive until 7:30 p.m., we have just lied. If we habitu-ally sin, our hearts will also condemn us. For our words of faith to possess strength, we must be fully persuaded and expectant. Jesus said, "Every city or house divided against itself will not stand" (Matt. 12:25). Paul described how Abraham took this posture, saying:

He did not waver at the promise of God through unbelief, but was strengthened in faith, giving glory to God, and being fully convinced that what He had promised He was also able to perform. And therefore "it was accounted to him for righteousness."

—ROMANS 4:20–22

Abraham was "fully convinced," yet most Christians are internally conflicted. It's not that they lack faith but that the enemy deceives them into giving up their confidence. Earlier we talked about how the enemy entices us to act outside of love, then condemns us for it. He does the same with faith. When we lie or speak idly, our spirits hear those words and will not agree with them because they are untrue or worthless. Our own hearts condemn us (1 John 3:20–21). This creates a division within us. The enemy then draws near and says, "You can't believe your own words because you are a liar and have no control over your tongue." The right response is for us to repent of the lies or idle words and regain confidence, but too many Christians simply lose faith and fall into condemnation, confusion, and doubt. In that condition they remain, disbelieving their own words, blaming themselves, not approaching God with boldness but rather cowering and cringing before Him.

The same happens when we sin in any area, but especially in the area of unforgiveness. In a unique way, unforgiveness can cause us to retain unbelief in our hearts. Jesus connected faith directly to forgiveness in Mark 11:23–26, and it is no coincidence that the most powerful faith message in the Bible is paired with a very pointed teaching on the subject of forgiveness. Immediately after Jesus said we would have whatever we ask for if we believe, He said, "And whenever you stand praying, if you have anything against anyone, forgive him, that your

Father in heaven may also forgive you your trespasses. But if you do not forgive, neither will your Father in heaven forgive your trespasses" (Mark 11:25–26).

This was one continuous teaching, yet so many people stop at the "faith" part and don't continue to the "forgiveness" part. Faith preachers are some of my favorite preachers, but many preach about getting a new home or new car but not nearly as much about how bitterness can short-circuit our faith. Like greed, sexual sin, jealousy, gossip, and more, failing to forgive constitutes agreement with Satan, which is faith in exactly the wrong direction. When we will not forgive, or when we persist in any sin, Satan attacks our faith with our record of wrongs, and in too many cases he takes people right out of the race. Their words become weak. Gone is the bold confidence they once had; distant are the greater works Jesus has for them to do.

The solution is simple: get back into the love walk, where faith, hope, and love operate in full strength. "A threefold cord is not quickly broken" (Eccles. 4:12). Get God's voice back into your voice. "The words that I speak to you are spirit, and they are life," Jesus said in John 6:63. Speak His words, become fully convinced of your righteousness through faith, repent, and get back to speaking with confidence and power.

Words Well Placed

The Bible tells us it makes a big difference not just what we say but how and when we say it. Colossians 4:6 says, "Let your speech always be with grace, seasoned with salt, that you may know how you ought to answer each one." And Proverbs 27:14 says, "He who blesses his friend with a loud voice, rising early in the morning, it will be counted a curse to him." Even a blessing can actually be a curse if spoken at the wrong time and at too great a volume!

"Pleasant words are like a honeycomb, sweetness to the soul and health to the bones," says Proverbs 16:24, and elsewhere, "A word fitly spoken is like apples of gold in settings of silver" (Prov. 25:11). These are beautiful descriptions of graceful speech "seasoned with salt." A word spoken clumsily or out of its proper time does not fit; it lacks impact. So our words of faith must be spoken rightly. It does no good to run our mouths off loudly and assertively and call it faith. No—faith includes graciousness, a sense of sweetness, and proper timing.

IT'S A FACT!

One research paper states that "only recently have psychologists started to find a connection between love languages and relationship satisfaction....It may be that when partners have different love languages, it's not enough to 'speak the other person's language'—you have to do it effectively and genuinely....Many couples in therapy report finding the idea of love languages very useful for learning how to better support and show love to each other."[9]

This is what Christian psychologist Gary Chapman was aiming at in identifying what he calls the five love languages. People appreciate different ways of expressing and receiving love, and it does not diminish our faith to "fitly" speak to someone in a well-considered way. In fact, it yields great benefits.

Fitly spoken faith words not only improve relationships, but also they lose none of their impact. "By long forbearance a ruler is persuaded, and a gentle tongue breaks a bone," says Proverbs

25:15, and "sweetness of speech increases persuasiveness" (Prov. 16:21, ESV). Our words gain force when we deliver them with the proper timing and tone.

The Proverbs also say, "The tongue of the wise uses knowledge rightly" (15:2), "the tongue of the wise promotes health" (12:18), and "a word spoken in due season, how good it is!" (15:23). To speak love words, we all have to work at transforming our speech. Taking 1 Corinthians 13:4–8 as our guide, we must speak patient and kind words; not envious, boastful words but humble ones. Not touchy, fretful, cranky, resentful, self-seeking words but only those that give life.

Oral Roberts used to say, "Something good is going to happen to me." And you know what? Something good always did! That kind of cultivated hope and verbalized faith get our thoughts aligned with God's thoughts. That's when confident, loving words of faith bubble up from our spirits and out of our mouths. These words are fitting and powerful. When we speak God's words, we speak with His voice. In 1 Corinthians 2:13 (NASB) Paul calls them "words [not] taught by human wisdom, but...those taught by the Spirit." The writer of Hebrews said, "The word of God is living and active, sharper than any two-edged sword, piercing to the division of soul and of spirit, of joints and of marrow, and discerning the thoughts and intentions of the heart" (Heb. 4:12, ESV).

We have this great responsibility and privilege of assigning our words to life-giving purposes. Think of it this way: You get to use your words to bless, build up, impart life, express love, give hope, and command healing by faith. You have the awesome calling to improve your family, your business, your ministry, your neighborhood, and every situation you are in with the power of spoken words.

Remember, thoughts not put into words will die unborn. Our faith, hope, and love must be verbalized to have any effect. The good result will come back on you too, because once we get our minds in line with God's, it breaks the control of negative thoughts. We simply do not believe the lies we used to fall for anymore.

Meditate on the Word of God day and night. Speak it to yourself and others. Listen to it in sermons, worship songs, and audio Bibles. Ponder it, mull it over, and let it go deep inside of you. It will be as Isaiah the prophet described:

> For as the rain comes down, and the snow from heaven, and do not return there, but water the earth, and make it bring forth and bud, that it may give seed to the sower and bread to the eater, so shall My word be that goes forth from My mouth; it shall not return to Me void, but it shall accomplish what I please, and it shall prosper in the thing for which I sent it. For you shall go out with joy, and be led out with peace; the mountains and the hills shall break forth into singing before you, and all the trees of the field shall clap their hands.
>
> —Isaiah 55:10–12

Prayer and Declarations

Father, thank You for the gift of supernaturally powerful "Spirit" words. Help me to use them in proper and effective ways, seasoning my speech with salt, sweetening it with graciousness, and strengthening it with softness when appropriate. Your Word never goes forth without effect, so I commit to speak Your words every day, in every circumstance—including when I am alone with You. Let Your words go forth through my mouth, by faith, with hope, and confident in love. Amen.

I will make every effort to speak kindly by faith.

My words are fitting and have their proper impact as I speak them at the right time and in the most excellent way.

I am able to change the way I speak and take charge over my mouth, allowing only words of life to proceed from it.

I repent for speaking idle, faithless words, and I commit to speaking kind, loving, encouraging, and faith-filled words.

I repent for speaking untruths because anything that undermines my confidence disempowers my words and causes my heart to condemn me.

CHAPTER 13

"A TSUNAMI OF LOVE"

THROUGHOUT THIS BOOK we've focused on the one thing that matters more than everything else when it comes to your life, your health, your well-being, and even your eternal destiny: love.

The ancient Greeks identified four types of love:

- phileo—friendship love
- storge—affectionate love between family members
- eros—sensual love
- agape—unconditional love (the God kind of love)

It is this last form of love, agape, that will change your life from the inside out, yet I believe most Christians have no concept of agape love. The word *love* is so misappropriated by the church and especially the world.

I love football.

I love ice cream.

I love pizza.

The Bible says, "He who does not love does not know God, for God is love" (1 John 4:8). And 1 Corinthians 13:4–8 lists all the different attributes or fruits of love. However, 1 John 3:18

213

says, "Let us not love in word or in tongue, but in deed and in truth." That means the God kind of love (agape) is shown by our actions. It is perhaps best demonstrated in the parable of the good Samaritan, found in Luke 10:30–37.

One day a lawyer stood up and tested Jesus, saying, "Teacher, what shall I do to inherit eternal life?" Jesus asked him, "What is written in the law?" The lawyer answered, "You shall love the LORD your God with all your heart, with all your soul, with all your strength, and with all your mind, and your neighbor as yourself" (v. 27). Remember, Jesus gave us a new love commandment, "to love one another as I have loved you" (John 13:34). The old love commandment was to love our neighbor as ourselves. This agape love is only possible by the Holy Spirit. (See Romans 5:5.) And Jesus said to him, "You have answered rightly; do this and you will live." The lawyer, wanting to justify himself, said to Jesus, "Who is my neighbor?" Jesus answered by telling him a story:

> "A certain man went down from Jerusalem to Jericho, and fell among thieves, who stripped him of his clothing, wounded him, and departed, leaving him half dead. Now by chance a certain priest came down that road. And when he saw him, he passed by on the other side. Likewise a Levite, when he arrived at the place, came and looked, and passed by on the other side. [Levites performed subordinate services associated with public worship, serving as musicians, gatekeepers, guardians, temple officials, etc.] But a certain Samaritan, as he journeyed, came where he was. And when he saw him, he had compassion. So he went to him and bandaged his wounds, pouring on oil and wine; and he set him on his own animal, brought him to an inn, and took care of him. On the next day, when he departed, he took out two denarii, gave them to the

innkeeper, and said to him, 'Take care of him; and whatever more you spend, when I come again, I will repay you.' So which of these three do you think was neighbor to him who fell among the thieves?" And he said, "He who showed mercy on him." Then Jesus said to him, "Go and do likewise."

This story is made all the more profound when you realize that the Jews of Jesus' day hated the Samaritans because the Samaritans rejected Jerusalem and its temple as sacred centers and believed that God chose Mount Gerizim in Samaria instead of Mount Zion in Jerusalem. However, both Jews and Samaritans worshipped Yahweh.

The Holy Spirit enables every Christian to demonstrate this agape love because the love of God has been poured out in our hearts by the Holy Spirit (Rom. 5:5).

STAMPED WITH THE KNOWLEDGE OF GOD

Author and pastor John Burke has researched near-death experiences (NDEs) over the last three decades. He has studied the commonalities of over one thousand people who have clinically died, been resuscitated, and claimed to experience life after death. Many medical doctors have been persuaded by the same evidence he found. Oncologist Jeffrey Long used to be an NDE skeptic, but after resuscitating over four thousand NDEs, he is no longer a skeptic but a believer in them. In Burke's book *Imagine the God of Heaven*, Dr. Long said, "NDEs provide such powerful scientific evidence that it is reasonable to accept the existence of an afterlife."[1]

NDE accounts demonstrate a consistent order of common events, including observing your resuscitation, traveling through a tunnel, and a life review in the presence of a God of light and love. Surveys in thirty-five countries indicate that millions have had an NDE, and many experience hell; 48 percent of NDEs experience a God of light and love, and 65 percent experience light that is love.[2]

Burke said he believes NDEs are God's gift to fill in with color the black-and-white words written in Scripture.[3] I have found that NDEs can provide some of the greatest evidence of agape love, or God's great love for all the people on the earth.

Howard Storm, a university professor who also experienced an NDE, described God's love this way: "Imagine all the love you've ever experienced…and put all that love across your lifetime into a single moment. Then multiply that by one thousand. That is God's love for you."[4]

People of all nationalities, professions, and backgrounds encounter the same God of light and love in their NDEs. God is not experienced as an impersonal force but as a personal God who knows each individual more intimately than they ever imagined. They all come back knowing that God is love and that love is what matters most to God.[5]

Jesus said in John 8:12, "I am the light of the world. Whoever follows me will never walk in darkness, but will have the light of life" (NIV).

Dr. Ron Smothermon was almost murdered by a friend who was housesitting for him. The house-sitter had stabbed him thirteen times in the chest, neck, and back with a nine-inch knife, and just as he was about to stab him in the heart, Dr. Smothermon had an NDE. A hallway appeared made of solid light. The light then exploded into a being and was brighter than the sun yet didn't hurt his eyes.

"It is not an ordinary light; it is a living being," Dr. Smothermon recalls. "…Instantly, the qualities of this person are written across my awareness....I am stamped with the knowledge of the nature of God....I never really understood that 'glory of God' thing before I witnessed it. God is truly glorious, magnificent, awesome, without equal. His glory is a light but made of infinite love. God's light appears like a sudden, silent, atomic bomb blast of white light, full of his power. Imagine being five feet away from the source of a nuclear explosion. But his light is more than light—it is overwhelming, a literal tsunami of infinite, unconditional love. All it touches transforms into perfect peace, and [it] blows away into irrelevancy any consideration about what is happening, replacing it with ineffable ecstasy, irresistible joy, love beyond comprehension—all in a singular package."[6]

Dr. Smothermon said this love (agape) is not an enhanced version of human love; it's love beyond our experiences, simply overpowering. It fills you with God's essence, and you know Him infinitely when your time comes to die, and it will—it is you and God swimming in an ocean of love. You become His love, and you are together in His light. Confronting God's love person to person inspires an intense desire to make His love known to every life form in the universe.

Miraculously, the attacker missed Dr. Smothermon's major nerves, arteries, and veins, and he went on to make a full recovery.

Wayne Fowler, an aerospace engineer and lawyer from Australia, suffered a painful heart attack. In his NDE, Wayne describes going into this presence, brighter than ten thousand suns. "At the center is the form of a man, arms outstretched toward me, like to welcome me and to hug me," Fowler says. "At that moment, I entered, I merged with the light, and the light merged with me. Like when Jesus said in John 17:21, 'I am

217

in you and you in me.' I was like a glass container being filled up, filled up with Him. I was experiencing the most ecstatic love. It was bliss beyond belief, rapture beyond reason, ecstasy beyond explanation, love times a billion, but our word *love* fails so badly. Imagine every loving relationship combined all together, then blow them all up billions of times all of that."[7]

Most of the NDE recipients report never having experienced love like that before, and their lives are usually radically changed. Many have an intense desire to make God's love known to others, but there are no words to adequately express that agape love. This God kind of love has been poured out in our hearts by the Holy Spirit in every believer (Rom. 5:5). As we meditate on love, practice love, and become doers of His Word as 1 John 3:18 says, let us not love in word or in tongue only, but in deeds and in truth. As this love grows, we too will radiate love and light because God is love.

Colossians 1:27 says, "To them God willed to make known what are the riches of the glory of this mystery among the Gentiles: which is Christ in you, the hope of glory." We need to get a revelation of the glorified, resurrected Jesus living in us and His love and light shining out of us—and then take this love and light to the world.

CONCLUSION

ABOVE ALL ELSE

MY FRIEND CHAD Bonk had a remarkable experience when he was a young pastor in Vancouver, Canada. At the time, he and his wife, Paula, had very little money, and their church was going through a terrible season of accusation and disintegration. Chad told me later it was the hardest time of their lives financially, spiritually, emotionally, and every other conceivable way.

While taking a few days away with Paula, Chad had an extraordinary supernatural encounter. Unexpectedly, an angel came into his room and said, "You have an appointment."

With that, Chad was transported to heaven, where he saw indescribably beautiful scenes of nature—perfect grass, water, sand, and animals, along with heavenly aromas and sounds. As he followed the angel, he saw he was being led to a man standing on the shore of a lake. The man was wearing a robe, and Chad took in every detail of his appearance. The man was skipping rocks and not doing a very good job of it.

"Hi, Chad," he said, then indicated his rock-skipping efforts and added, "I haven't done this very often."

It was the apostle Paul.

In the ensuing conversation Chad was astonished to find that

Paul knew everything about his life—details about his family, where he was going to live in the future, and much more. Chad climbed onto a big boulder on the lakeshore and sat while Paul talked to him for a long time. The main thing he talked about was loving people. The biggest problem in the church worldwide, Paul said, was that Christians had forgotten how to love people in the world. Attention was focused instead on building nice physical structures and feeding those who had heard the same message a thousand times. Jesus came to love the unlovable, but so many churches are simply loving those already in the body.

Another major problem, Paul said, is that Christians don't know how to love their own brothers and sisters. Christians persecute each other and inflict painful wounds within churches. Self-centeredness and agenda-seeking have taken the place of loving one another.

Third, pastors have forgotten how to love people. The goal of any ministry, Paul said, is first and foremost to love people, no matter if you are a pastor, a prophet, an evangelist, an apostle, or a teacher.

There was much more to Chad's life-changing encounter, which he is writing in a book. He told me, "[Paula and I] had to get torn down to the foundations so we had nothing else to rely on because God had a divine call on our lives." As his friend and doctor, I can tell you Chad's call is real—and so is the message of love he brought back from Paul in that heavenly experience. It directs me again to how critical it is to love God and love each other above all else.

Words to Live By

In the middle of writing this book, Mary and I traveled to my alma mater, Oral Roberts University, in Tulsa, Oklahoma, to see my daughter-in-law, Meredith, graduate with her master's degree in Christian counseling. She now has a Christian counseling practice in Southlake, Texas. In a packed Mabee Center, the overflow crowd gave high praise and worship to God, led by a full choir and band. In attendance was a very enthusiastic assembly of parents, students, professors, staff, dignitaries, and loved ones from all over America. The energy in the room was far beyond what we were expecting from a normal graduation service, and we knew God was present in a special way.

When keynote speaker Rick Warren got up to speak, things went to a whole other level. Rick is the founding pastor of Saddleback Church and one of the best-selling authors of all time. His book *The Purpose-Driven Life* is read around the world and has sold millions of copies.

Rick started by sharing an experience he had with Oral Roberts personally, one which he had never shared publicly until that day.

> When Oral and Evelyn retired, they moved to Newport Beach, California, which is my area....[One night] I had the chance to ask Oral a question that I had asked another dear friend of mine, John Wimber. I once asked John, "When you pray for people being healed, what is the most important thing going through your mind as you're praying for the healing of someone's body?" I asked that question of Oral, and interestingly enough, he said the exact same four words that John Wimber had told me probably five years earlier. He said this: "That people feel loved. That people feel loved."

...As a pastor...I have stood at the bedside of maybe thousands of people as they took their last breath. What people say in their final moments is pretty important. They don't mess around, when people are dying, in their last words. Nobody has ever said, "Pastor Rick, bring me my trophies. I want to look at them one more time." Or even, "Bring me my college graduation certificate. I want to look at it one more time." When people are dying and they know their time is short, what they want in the room is not things or trophies or achievement; what they want are the people they love.

We all eventually figure out that it's all about love. It's all about relationships. I just pray you will figure it out a whole lot sooner, that it's not about achievement; that it's not about fame; that it's not about fortune; that it's not about all the things that you dream of accomplishing in life. Those are great goals, but Paul says, "Without love I am nothing. I am a sounding brass and a tinkling cymbal. If I have not love, I'm nothing."

...You see, you were made by God and you were made for God, and until you figure that out, life is never going to make sense. The Bible says, "God is love." It doesn't say He has love. It says He is love. Love is the essence of God. It is the nature of God. It's who God is. God is love! The only reason there is any love in the universe is because our Creator is a loving God. If God was not a God of love, there would be no love in the universe. The only reason you have the ability to give love and to receive love is because you were made in God's image....God is love and He gave you the ability to love Him and to be loved back. He gave you the ability to love others.

Your first purpose in life is not to love God. It is to let God love you. The Bible says, "We love because He first loved us." We respond to the love of God. I can't tell you in my lifetime how many people have come up to me and said something like, "You know, Rick, I think my problem is I just don't love God enough." And I say, "That's not your problem. Your problem is you don't understand how much He loves you, because if you understood how much God loves you, you can't help but love Him. When you understand [that] and...you finally feel loved by God, unconditionally loved by God, it changes you."[1]

RECOMMENDED SUPPLEMENTS

WHILE THIS BOOK is designed to help you achieve optimum spiritual health, I want you to have access to the following supplements for a holistic approach to your wellness: body, mind, and spirit.

SUPPLEMENTS

Divine Health supplements
Available at shop.drcolbert.com or by calling (407) 732-6952

- Divine Health High Potency Turmeric with Bioperine—contains 500 mg per capsule of active curcuminoids (active compound), 5 mg of bioperine, and 500 mg of sunflower lecithin for improved absorption. It supports healthy brain function and a healthy immune response and provides joint and inflammation support.

- Divine Health NAD Powder—contains nicotinamide riboside chloride powder. It supports natural energy production (not caffeine) and supports focus and attention. It also supports healthy brain function and healthy brain aging.

- Divine Health Pickle Powder—contains curcumin 1,000 mg of 95% active curcuminoids, ginger 1,000 mg, and the active form of Boswellia 300 mg. It also contains the electrolytes calcium, sodium, magnesium, and potassium, which aids in the prevention of muscle cramps and promotes hydration. It also contains bioperine 50 mg for improved absorption. It supports joints and recovery from strenuous exercise and provides support for inflammation. It was initially developed for pickleball players but is excellent for all participants in sports, especially if forty years of age or older.

- Fiber Zone—great-tasting psyllium husk powder with prebiotics (inulin); available flavors: lemon-lime and berry (contains soluble and insoluble fibers; I often recommend 1–2 scoops daily)

- Enhanced Multivitamin—contains the active forms of vitamins, including B vitamins, with chelated minerals for better absorption of the minerals

- Organic Green Supremefood—superfood drink with fourteen organic fermented veggies and grasses and no nightshades, with four different strains of probiotics and four digestive enzymes. It is fermented for better digestion and less gas.

- Organic Red Supremefood—contains nine organic fruits and is low sugar and includes raspberry, blueberry, cranberry, acai, and pomegranate

- Collagen powder—hydrolyzed collagen consists of chicken collagen, containing Type I and Type II collagen. As you age, your body slowly loses collagen throughout the body (hair, nails, joints, bones, heart, and skin). Your body's joints and skin repair at night, so it's best to take ½ to 1 scoop in any liquid thirty minutes before bed. Available in chocolate, vanilla, and unflavored.

- Divine Health Biotics—a powerful probiotic to help restore a leaky gut; contains Bifidobacterium breve, Bifidobacterium lactis, Lactobacillus plantarum, Bacillus coagulans, Bacillus subtilis, and the prebiotics fructooligosaccharides (FOS), and galactooligosaccharides (GOS). One veggie capsule contains sixteen billion CFUs (colony forming units) and 200 mg of prebiotics.

- Brain Zone Basic—includes the active forms of the B vitamins—including methylated folate, methylcobalamin, and pyridoxal 5-phosphate in optimal dosages—curcumin, and TMG (trimethyl glycine) to lower homocysteine levels. (I especially recommend this for people with the MTHFR gene mutation and for patients with an elevated homocysteine level.)

- Divine Health Carb Assist—a new supplement that supports healthy blood sugar levels by improving carbohydrate metabolism, insulin sensitivity, and the processing of dietary carbohydrates

- Super Vitamin K2—contains high-dose vitamin K2, 200 mg per capsule, consisting of MK-7 for better bioavailability. Vitamin K2 regulates calcium metabolism in the body, helping to build strong bones and preventing calcium buildup in the arteries, including cerebral arteries, thus supporting good blood flow to the brain.

- Divine Health Nano Glutathione—Glutathione is a powerful antioxidant often called "the master antioxidant" that combats inflammation, oxidative stress, infections, mental stress, toxins, and heavy metals in the body. Glutathione levels are being depleted by aging, toxin overload, poor diet, and stressed lifestyles. Nanotechnology offers rapid and more complete absorption from the GI tract.

- Q10 Vital—contains 100 mg of CoQ10, which is a crucial antioxidant for providing energy to all cells in the body. It is especially important for optimal cardiovascular health.

- Divine Health Sleep Ease—contains natural supplements including GABA, magnesium glycinate, 5-HTP (5-hydroxytryptophan), L-theanine, melatonin, lemon balm extract, and ashwagandha, which helps one fall asleep and stay asleep.

Other recommended supplement

- Vitamin D3 Chocolate Chew—2,000 international units (IU)

To book an appointment with Dr. Colbert, call (407) 331-7007. Follow him on YouTube at Dr. Don Colbert MD, and tune into his podcast, *Divine Health with Dr. Don Colbert*, on the Charisma Podcast Network.

A PERSONAL NOTE FROM DON COLBERT, MD

God desires to heal you of disease. His Word is full of promises that confirm His love for you and His desire to give you His abundant life. His desire includes more than physical health for you; He wants to make you whole in your mind and spirit as well as through a personal relationship with His Son, Jesus Christ.

If you haven't met my best friend, Jesus, I would like to take this opportunity to introduce you to Him. It is very simple. If you are ready to let Him come into your life and become your best friend, all you need to do is sincerely pray this prayer:

Lord Jesus, I want to know You as my Savior and Lord. I believe and confess out loud that You are the Son of God and that You died for my sins. I also believe and confess that You were raised from the dead and now sit at the right hand of the Father praying for me. I ask You to forgive me for my sins, and I invite You into my heart so I can be Your child and live with You eternally. Thank You for Your peace. Help me to walk

with You so I can begin to know You as my best friend
and my Lord. Amen.

If you have prayed this prayer, you have just made the most important decision of your life. I rejoice with you in your decision and your new relationship with Jesus. Please contact my publisher at pray4me@charismamedia.com so that we can send you some materials that will help you become established in your relationship with the Lord. We look forward to hearing from you.

NOTES

Introduction

1. Molly Carman and David Closson, "New Barna Research Reveals Extent of America's Loss of Faith," June 22, 2021, https://www.frc.org/blog/2021/06/new-barna-research-reveals-extent-americas-loss-faith.

2. Carman and Closson, "New Barna Research Reveals Extent of America's Loss of Faith."

3. Carman and Closson, "New Barna Research Reveals Extent of America's Loss of Faith."

4. "The US Luxury Boom 2024," YouGov, April 23, 2024, https://business.yougov.com/content/49189-us-luxury-shoppers-report-2024.

Chapter 1

1. Kenneth D. Kochanek et al., "Mortality in the United States, 2022," National Center for Health Statistics Data Brief No. 492, March 2024, https://www.cdc.gov/nchs/products/databriefs/db492.htm.

2. Tobias Esch and George B. Stefano, "Love Promotes Health," *Neuro Endocrinology Letters* 26, no. 3 (June 2005): 264–7, https://pubmed.ncbi.nlm.nih.gov/15990734/; Tobias Esch, "The Significance of Stress for the Cardiovascular System: Stress-Associated Cardiovascular Diseases and Non-Pharmaceutical Therapy Options," *Apotheken Magazin* 21 (2003): 8–15; Tobias Esch et al., "The Therapeutic Use of the Relaxation Response in Stress-Related Diseases," *Medical Science Monitor* 9, no. 2 (2003): RA23–RA34, https://pubmed.ncbi.nlm.nih.gov/12601303/; Tobias Esch et al., "Commonalities in the Central Nervous

System's Involvement with Complementary Medical Therapies: Limbic Morphinergic Processes," *Medical Science Monitor* 10, no. 6 (2004): MS6–MS17, https://www.researchgate.net/publication/8532503_Commonalities_in_the_central_nervous_system's_involvement_with_complementary_medical_therapies_Limbic_morphinergic_processes; Tobias Esch and George B. Stefano, "The Neurobiology of Pleasure, Reward Processes, Addiction, and Their Health Implications," *Neuro Endocrinology Letters* 25, no. 4 (August 2004): 235–51, https://pubmed.ncbi.nlm.nih.gov/15361811/.

3. Charlie Huntington and Tchiki Davis, "Why Love Is Good for Well-Being: Discover How It Contributes to Your Well-Being and How to Cultivate More Love," *Psychology Today*, updated January 9, 2024, https://www.psychologytoday.com/intl/blog/click-here-for-happiness/202304/why-love-is-good-for-well-being; William J. Chopik, "Associations Among Relational Values, Support, Health, and Well-Being Across the Adult Lifespan," *Personal Relationships* 24, no. 2 (2017): 408–422, https://onlinelibrary.wiley.com/doi/full/10.1111/pere.12187. See also Eva Kahana et al., "Loving Others: The Impact of Compassionate Love on Later-Life Psychological Well-Being," *The Journals of Gerontology: Series B* 76, no. 2 (February 2021): 391–402, https://doi.org/10.1093/geronb/gbaa188.

4. C. Sue Carter and Stephen W. Porges, "The Biochemistry of Love: An Oxytocin Hypothesis," *Science & Society* 14 (2012): 12–16, https://doi.org/10.1038/embor.2012.191.

5. Daniel Cox et al., "How Prevalent Is Pornography?," Institute for Family Studies, May 3, 2022, https://ifstudies.org/blog/how-prevalent-is-pornography.

6. Julianne Holt-Lunstad et al., "Social Relationships and Mortality Risk: A Meta-Analytic Review," *PLOS Medicine* 7, no. 7 (July 27, 2010): e1000316, https://www.ncbi.nlm.nih.gov/pmc/articles/PMC2910600/.

7. Holt-Lunstad et al., "Social Relationships and Mortality Risk."

8. Eric W. Dolan, "The Psychology of Love: 10 Groundbreaking Insights into the Science of Relationships," PsyPost, February 14, 2024, https://www.psypost.org/the-psychology-of-love-10-groundbreaking-insights-into-the-science-of-relationships/.

CHAPTER 2

1. Mayo Clinic staff, "Forgiveness: Letting Go of Grudges and Bitterness," Mayo Clinic, accessed September 10, 2024, https://www.mayoclinic.org/healthy-lifestyle/adult-health/in-depth/forgiveness/art-20047692.

CHAPTER 3

1. T. L. Osborn, *The Power of Positive Desire: Seven Vital Principles for Unlimited Living* (Harrison House, 2005), 59.

2. Kenneth E. Hagin, *Love: The Way to Victory* (Faith Library Publications, 1975), 52.

3. Linda Nevin, "Unlocking the Healing Power of Love: The Link Between Love and Physical Health," LindaNevin.com, May 16, 2023, https://www.lindanevin.com/post/the-surprising-link-between-love-and-physical-health-a-guide-to-unlocking-the-healing-power-of-love.

4. Kahana et al., "Loving Others," 391–402.

5. R. F. Baumeister and M. R. Leary, "The Need to Belong: Desire for Interpersonal Attachments as a Fundamental Human Motivation," *Psychological Bulletin* 117, no. 3 (May 1995): 497–529, https://pubmed.ncbi.nlm.nih.gov/7777651/.

6. Eva Kahana et al., "Altruism, Helping, and Volunteering: Pathways to Well-Being in Late Life," *Journal of Aging Health* 25, no. 1 (February 2013): 159–87, https://pubmed.ncbi.nlm.nih.gov/23324536/.

CHAPTER 4

1. Jamie Ducharme, "5 Ways Love Is Good for Your Health," *Time*, February 14, 2018, https://time.com/5136409/health-benefits-love/.

2. Holt-Lunstad et al., "Social Relationships and Mortality Risk."

3. Jeffrey Kluger, "5 Ways Loneliness Can Hurt Your Health," *Time*, November 13, 2017, https://time.com/5009202/loneliness-effects/.

4. Ducharme, "5 Ways Love Is Good for Your Health."

5. Ducharme, "5 Ways Love Is Good for Your Health."

6. Bible Hub, s.v. "*hallomai*," accessed September 10, 2024, https://biblehub.com/greek/242.htm.

7. "Annual Prevalence of Use of Adderall for Grades 8, 10, and 12 from 2009 to 2022," Statista, accessed September 10, 2024, https://www.statista.com/statistics/696590/us-annual-prevalence-of-adderall-use-in-grades-8-10-12-since-2009/; "Data and Statistics on ADHD," U.S. Centers for Disease Control and Prevention, accessed September 10, 2024, https://www.cdc.gov/adhd/data/?CDC_AAref_Val=https://www.cdc.gov/ncbddd/adhd/data.html.

8. "Annual Prevalence of Use of Adderall for Grades 8, 10, and 12 from 2009 to 2022," Statista; "Data and Statistics on ADHD," U.S. Centers for Disease Control and Prevention.

9. R. Buckminster Fuller, *Critical Path* (St. Martin's Press, 1981).

10. Ravi Jasti, "How AI in Business Intelligence Redefines the Typical Business User," *Forbes*, July 28, 2023, https://www.forbes.com/sites/forbestechcouncil/2023/07/28/how-ai-in-business-intelligence-redefines-the-typical-business-user/, emphasis added.

11. Osborn, *The Power of Positive Desire*, 189–190.

12. Osborn, *The Power of Positive Desire*, 191–192.

13. Osborn, *The Power of Positive Desire*, 170.

14. Judah Schiller, "Average Human Attention Span by Age: 31 Statistics," The Treetop (ABA Therapy), July 17, 2024, https://www.thetreetop.com/statistics/average-human-attention-span.

CHAPTER 5

1. Osborn, *The Power of Positive Desire*, 90–91.

2. R. A. Emmons, *Thanks! How the New Science of Gratitude Can Make You Happier* (Houghton Mifflin Harcourt, 2007).

3. Emmons, *Thanks!*

4. Emmons, *Thanks!*

5. R. A. Emmons and M. E. McCullough, "Counting Blessings Versus Burdens: An Experimental Investigation of Gratitude and Subjective Well-Being in Daily Life," *Journal of Personality and Social Psychology* 84, no. 2 (2003): 377–389, https://doi.org/10.1037/0022-3514.84.2.377.

6. Eric W. Dolan, "The Psychology of Love: 10 Groundbreaking Insights into the Science of Relationships," PsyPost, February 14, 2024, https://www.psypost.org/the-psychology-of-love-10-groundbreaking-insights-into-the-science-of-relationships/.

CHAPTER 6

1. Fred Luskin, *Forgive for Good: A Proven Prescription for Health and Happiness* (HarperOne, 2002), xv.

2. Luskin, *Forgive for Good.*

3. Luskin, *Forgive for Good.*

4. Alex H. S. Harris et al., "Effects of a Group Forgiveness Intervention on Forgiveness, Perceived Stress, and Trait-Anger," *Journal of Clinical Psychology* 62, no. 6 (2006): 715–733, https://onlinelibrary.wiley.com/doi/10.1002/jclp.20264.

5. Gail Ironson et al., "An Increase in Religiousness/Spirituality Occurs After HIV Diagnosis and Predicts Slower Disease Progression over 4 Years in People with HIV," *Journal of General Internal Medicine* 21, suppl. 5 (2006): S62–68, https://link.springer.com/article/10.1111/j.1525-1497.2006.00648.x#citeas.

6. Bryan Robinson, "New Study Shows the Mental and Physical Harm of Holding Workplace Grudges," *Forbes*, February 5,

2022, https://www.forbes.com/sites/bryanrobinson/2022/02/05/
new-study-shows-the-mental-and-physical-harm-of-holding-
workplace-grudges/?sh=1671964945f8.

7. Shoba Sreenlvasan and Linda E. Weinberger, "Forever Resentful:
Grudges Are Easy to Develop but Hard to Let Go," *Psychology
Today*, September 26, 2023, https://www.psychologytoday.com/
us/blog/emotional-nourishment/202309/forever-resentful-
grudges-are-easy-to-develop-but-hard-to-let-go.

8. Sreenlvasan and Weinberger, "Forever Resentful; Robinson,
"New Study Shows the Mental and Physical Harm of Holding
Workplace Grudges."

9. Sreenlvasan and Weinberger, "Forever Resentful."

10. Sreenlvasan and Weinberger, "Forever Resentful."

11. Mother Teresa, *Where There Is Love, There Is God* (Doubleday,
2010), 65.

CHAPTER 7

1. Myung-Sun Chung, "Relation Between Lack of Forgiveness
and Depression: The Moderating Effect of Self-Compassion,"
Psychological Reports 119, no. 3 (December 2016): 573–585,
https://pubmed.ncbi.nlm.nih.gov/27511966/.

2. Yun-Zi Liu et al., "Inflammation: The Common Pathway of
Stress-Related Diseases," *Frontiers in Human Neuroscience* 11
(June 2017), https://doi.org/10.3389/fnhum.2017.00316.

3. Markham Heid, "How Stress Affects Cancer Risk," MD
Anderson Cancer Center, December 2014, https://www.
mdanderson.org/publications/focused-on-health/how-stress-
affects-cancer-risk.h21-1589046.html.

4. Kara E. Hannibal and Mark D. Bishop, "Chronic Stress, Cortisol
Dysfunction, and Pain: A Psychoneuroendocrine Rationale for
Stress Management in Pain Rehabilitation," *Physical Therapy*
94, no. 12 (December 2014): 1816–1825, https://doi.org/10.2522/
ptj.20130597.

5. Karen A. Scott et al., "Effects of Chronic Social Stress on Obesity," *Etiology of Obesity* 1 (January 2012): 16–25, https://doi.org/10.1007/s13679-011-0006-3.

6. Luskin, *Forgive for Good.*

7. Dodie Osteen, *Healed of Cancer* (John Osteen Publications, 1986), 17.

8. Robinson, "New Study Shows the Mental and Physical Harm of Holding Workplace Grudges."

9. Hannibal and Bishop, "Chronic Stress, Cortisol Dysfunction, and Pain."

10. Jody Louise Davis et al., "Forgiveness and Health in Nonmarried Dyadic Relationships," chapter in *Forgiveness and Health*, eds., Loren Toussaint, Everett Worthington, and David R. Williams (Springer Dordrecht, 2015), 239–253.

11. Katia G. Reinert, "The Influence of Forgiveness on Health and Healing," *Journal of Family Research and Practice* 1, no. 1 (July 2021): 87–97, https://www.academia.edu/87516855/The_Influence_of_Forgiveness_on_Health_and_Healing.

12. Andrea Danese and Bruce S. McEwen, "Adverse Childhood Experiences, Allostasis, Allostatic Load, and Age-Related Disease," *Physiology and Behavior* 106, no. 1 (April 12, 2012): 29–39, https://doi.org/10.1016/j.physbeh.2011.08.019; Reinert, "The Influence of Forgiveness on Health and Healing."

13. Katia G. Reinert et al., "The Role of Religious Involvement in the Relationship Between Early Trauma and Health Outcomes Among Adult Survivors," *Journal of Child and Adolescent Trauma* 9 (2016): 231–241, https://link.springer.com/article/10.1007/s40653-015-0067-7. See also Reinert, "The Influence of Forgiveness on Health and Healing."

14. Reinert, "The Influence of Forgiveness on Health and Healing."

15. Loren L. Toussaint and Everett L. Worthington Jr., "Forgiveness," *The Psychologist* 30 (July 3, 2017): 28–33, https://thepsychologist.

bps.org.uk/volume-30/august-2017/forgiveness. See also Reinert, "The Influence of Forgiveness on Health and Healing."

16. Corrie ten Boom, *Tramp for the Lord* (Jove Books, 1978), 57.

17. Kirsten Weir, "Forgiveness Can Improve Mental and Physical Health: Research Shows How to Get There," *Monitor on Psychology* 48, no. 1 (January 2017): 30, https://www.apa.org/monitor/2017/01/ce-corner.

18. Weir, "Forgiveness Can Improve Mental and Physical Health."

19. Weir, "Forgiveness Can Improve Mental and Physical Health."

20. Weir, "Forgiveness Can Improve Mental and Physical Health."

21. Weir, "Forgiveness Can Improve Mental and Physical Health."

22. Weir, "Forgiveness Can Improve Mental and Physical Health."

CHAPTER 8

1. Luskin, *Forgive for Good*, 80.

2. Hagin, *Love: The Way to Victory*, 152.

3. Hagin, *Love: The Way to Victory*, 186.

4. Ducharme, "5 Ways Love Is Good for Your Health."

5. "Compared to 20 or 30 Years Ago, Do You Think People Are More Rude, Less Rude, or About the Same?," Statista, accessed September 10, 2024, https://www.statista.com/statistics/539628/rudeness-survey-united-states.

6. Katelyn N. G. Long et al., "Forgiveness of Others and Subsequent Health and Well-Being in Mid-Life: A Longitudinal Study on Female Nurses," *BMC Psychology* 8, no. 104 (2020), https://doi.org/10.1186/s40359-020-00470-w.

7. Ironson et al., "An Increase in Religiousness/Spirituality Occurs After HIV Diagnosis and Predicts Slower Disease Progression over 4 Years in People with HIV."

8. Liu et al., "Inflammation."

9. Heid, "How Stress Affects Cancer Risk."

10. G. L. Reed and R. D. Enright, "The Effects of Forgiveness Therapy on Depression, Anxiety, and Posttraumatic Stress for Women After Spousal Emotional Abuse," *Journal of Consulting and Clinical Psychology* 74, no. 5 (2006): 920–929, https://doi.org/10.1037/0022-006X.74.5.920.

11. Weir, "Forgiveness Can Improve Mental and Physical Health."

12. Nathaniel G. Wade et al., "Efficacy of Psychotherapeutic Interventions to Promote Forgiveness: A Meta-Analysis," *Journal of Consulting and Clinical Psychology* 82, no. 1 (2014): 154–170, https://doi.org/10.1037/a0035268; Weir, "Forgiveness Can Improve Mental and Physical Health."

13. Weir, "Forgiveness Can Improve Mental and Physical Health."

14. Weir, "Forgiveness Can Improve Mental and Physical Health."

Chapter 9

1. Martin E. P. Seligman, *Learned Optimism: How to Change Your Mind and Your Life* (Vintage, 2006), 81.

2. Samuel J. Abrams, "Americans Are More Optimistic Than You Think," Survey Center on American Life, March 14, 2022, https://www.americansurveycenter.org/americans-are-more-optimistic-than-you-think/.

3. Seligman, *Learned Optimism*, 7.

4. Seligman, *Learned Optimism*, 4–5 (emphasis added).

5. Seligman, *Learned Optimism*, 8, 16.

6. Luskin, *Forgive for Good*, 86.

7. Luskin, *Forgive for Good*, 86.

8. Mikko Pänkäläinen et al., "Pessimism and Risk of Death from Coronary Heart Disease Among Middle-Aged and Older Finns: An Eleven-Year Follow-Up Study," *BMC Public Health* 16, no. 1124 (2016), https://doi.org/10.1186/s12889-016-3764-8.

9. "The New Science of Optimism and Longevity," excerpted from Immaculata De Vivo and Daniel Lumera, *The Biology of Kindness* (MIT Press, 2024).

10. De Vivo and Lumera, *The Biology of Kindness*.

11. Luskin, *Forgive for Good*, 86.

12. Luskin, *Forgive for Good*, 86.

13. Luskin, *Forgive for Good*, 86.

14. Seligman, *Learned Optimism*, 175.

15. Seligman, *Learned Optimism*, 16.

16. Seligman, *Learned Optimism*, 44.

17. Seligman, *Learned Optimism*, 49.

18. Seligman, *Learned Optimism*, 47–48.

19. Seligman, *Learned Optimism*, 45.

20. Seligman, *Learned Optimism*, 44.

21. Seligman, *Learned Optimism*, 137 (bracketed comment added).

22. Seligman, *Learned Optimism*, 44 (bracketed comment added).

23. Mother Teresa, *Where There Is Love, There Is God*, 64–65.

24. *Britannica*, s.v. "Korean Air Lines Flight 007," accessed September 10, 2024, https://www.britannica.com/event/Korean-Air-Lines-flight-007.

25. Seligman, *Learned Optimism*, 207.

CHAPTER 10

1. De Vivo and Lumera, *The Biology of Kindness*.

2. Jenna Lee and Mark V. Pellegrini, *Biochemistry, Telomere, and Telomerase* (StatPearls Publishing, 2022).

3. De Vivo and Lumera, *The Biology of Kindness*.

4. Seligman, *Learned Optimism*, 14.

5. Seligman, *Learned Optimism*, 175.

6. Seligman, *Learned Optimism*, 175.

7. Seligman, *Learned Optimism*, 16.

8. Osteen, *Healed of Cancer*, 54–55.

9. "The New Science of Optimism and Longevity," excerpted from Immaculata De Vivo and Daniel Lumera, *The Biology of Kindness* (MIT Press, 2024).

10. Seligman, *Learned Optimism*, 89–90.

11. Seligman, Learned Optimism, 220.

12. De Vivo and Lumera, *The Biology of Kindness*.

13. Seligman, *Learned Optimism*, 175.

14. Seligman, *Learned Optimism*, 221.

15. Seligman, *Learned Optimism*, 91.

16. Robert A. Emmons and Robin Stern, "Gratitude as a Psychotherapeutic Intervention," *Journal of Clinical Psychology* 69, no. 8 (2013): 846–855, https://onlinelibrary.wiley.com/doi/10.1002/jclp.22020; Emmons and McCullough, "Counting Blessings Versus Burdens."

17. Emmons and McCullough, "Counting Blessings Versus Burdens."

18. Michael E. McCullough et al., "The Grateful Disposition: A Conceptual and Empirical Topography," *Journal of Personality and Social Psychology* 82, no. 1 (2002): 112–127.

19. Marti Pieper, "How Andrew Wommack's Son Moved From Morgue to Miracle," Charisma News, April 19, 2021, https://charismanews.com/marketplace/how-andrew-wommack-s-son-moved-from-morgue-to-miracle/.

20. Osborn, *The Power of Positive Desire*, 76.

21. Osborn, *The Power of Positive Desire*, 73.

22. Osborn, *The Power of Positive Desire*, 100.

23. Osborn, *The Power of Positive Desire*, 130–132.

24. Osborn, *The Power of Positive Desire*, 155.

CHAPTER 11

1. Osborn, *The Message That Works*, 285.
2. Osborn, *The Message That Works*, 245.
3. Osborn, *The Message That Works*, 231.
4. Mother Teresa, *Where There Is Love, There Is God*, 80.

CHAPTER 12

1. Osteen, *Healed of Cancer*, 58–59.
2. Osteen, *Healed of Cancer*, 58–59.
3. Osteen, *Healed of Cancer*, 15.
4. Osteen, *Healed of Cancer*, 26–27.
5. Osteen, *Healed of Cancer*, 59–60.
6. Osteen, *Healed of Cancer*, 21.
7. Osteen, *Healed of Cancer*, 32, 57, 59–60.
8. Osborn, *The Power of Positive Desire*, 162.
9. Huntington and Davis, "Why Love Is Good for Well-Being."

CHAPTER 13

1. John Burke, *Imagine the God of Heaven* (Tyndale, 2023), 24.
2. Burke, *Imagine the God of Heaven*, 31.
3. Burke, *Imagine the God of Heaven*, 24, 63.
4. Burke, *Imagine the God of Heaven*, 18.
5. Burke, *Imagine the God of Heaven*, 19.
6. Burke, *Imagine the God of Heaven*, 60–61.
7. Burke, *Imagine the God of Heaven*, 91–92.

CONCLUSION

1. Oral Roberts University, "Graduation 2024 Commencement Address: Rick Warren," YouTube, May 10, 2024, 21:20, https://www.youtube.com/watch?v=TJ4K5WFWIuw.

MY FREE GIFT TO YOU

Dear Reader

As my way of spreading God's love,

I am offering the eBook version of
Dr. Colbert's Health Zone Essentials
to you for FREE!

God Bless Your Abundant Heart,

Dr. Don Colbert

SILOAM